Let's Get Naked

The Sexy Activity Book for Couples

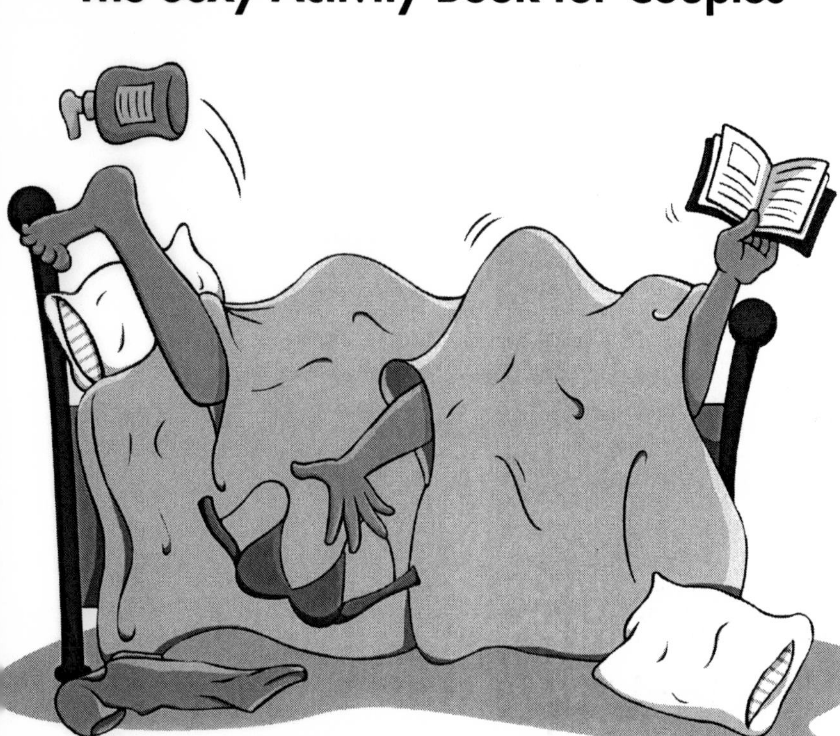

Design & Illustrations by Robyn Durst
First Edition

Published by Neuron Publishing
www.neuronpublishing.com
www.LoveBookOnline.com

Let's Get Naked

The Sexy Activity Book for Couples

Warning!

Let me begin by saying that this book is meant to be for adult "sexy fun time". In no way am I suggesting, instructing or demanding you to go out there and get your freak on irresponsibly. I am not a sexpert, sex psychologist, or even good at sex in general.

This book is obviously meant for grown adults, so if you're under the age of 18, put it down right now. I mean it, young man (or young lady). You will be in serious trouble. I'll wait.

I'm not an idiot. I know that you haven't put the book down yet, so Mom, don't blame me if junior gets caught with this book.

Also, because my lawyer told me to fully protect myself, I have to state the following:

- Use protection: don't yell at me if there's any unplanned pregnancies, unintended diseases, or unwelcomed accidents on your new carpeting.

- Be responsible: don't be a dummy and try these games in public, at work, or with someone who isn't a consenting adult. I can't be held responsible if you get arrested, fired, or slapped in the face.

Okay, I think I've covered everything. Just in case I haven't, the next page consists of general "lawyer-y" fine print to make sure I've covered my ass:

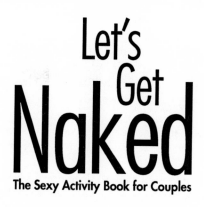

The fine print (damn, print, you FINE!): *you can roll your eyes now

I cannot be held responsible for anything that happens to you, to other people, to your dog, cat, hamster or goldfish, to yours or other's property, to the mailman, or to your existing or future children while using this book or doing anything that resides in it.

I cannot be blamed for what your mom says or does when she finds out you have this book.

I think I'm pretty funny, even though deep down I know I'm not. But I try anyway. That said, there are some very obvious jokes in this book. I can't be held responsible if you're stupid and actually try some of the "optional things you need" that I joke about, such as utilizing a hamster in any of these games. Please, don't do anything with any hamsters. Seriously, don't.

I like cheese.

If you thought that this page would contain serious, legal jargon then I assume you probably haven't read it. Too bad for you. I have a friend who can predict the future, and he says that these will be the winning lotto numbers for next week's drawing: 12 22 34 45 67.

If you have read this far, and intend on playing those numbers, chances are you won't win. I do not have a friend who can predict the future. I don't even have friends. But, if you do play them and win, congrats! And I expect you'll share some of your fortune with me. Please? I could really use the money.

Okay, you sillies, enough of my lame attempt at humor. If you wanted a book that would actually make you laugh, you should have bought a real comedian's biography, like Gerald McBillingsly's. Don't know who Gerald McBillingsly is? Neither do I. I can't use a real comedian's name or else I'll get sued. So I made him up. Any resemblance to any persons living or dead is pure coincidence. Boo-yah.

No, I do not have brain damage.

Now, go have fun playing these games!

Table of Contents

Table of Contents Cont.

Psssst, see that icon to the left? That's our little "tips" icon. Cheeky, I know. I scattered these throughout the book to indicate sexy tips for intimate, romantic or just plain dirty things to do to ramp up your passion. So when you see these, read them and impress your partner with a new move.

How to use this book

There's no right or wrong way to use this book. Flip to a game you want to try, play each game page by page, or just open the book randomly and play that game.

Just make sure you have fun while doing them.

You can use this book to spice up your love life, to get to know your partner a little better, or to learn some new sex stuff that you were unaware of!

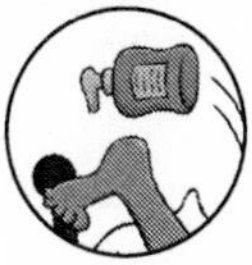

Foreplay

If you're unsure of what that word means, I suggest your partner find a new lover.

Is that too harsh? Okay, I suggest your partner lower their standards. Better?

Seriously, this section includes games that'll get you in the mood. That's the intent, anyways.

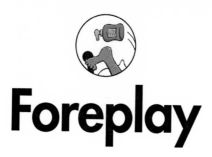

What's Your Porn Persona?

What you need:

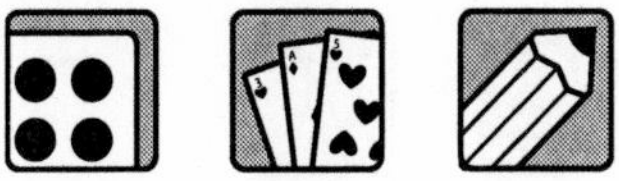

A Die -or- Cards Ace-6 Pencil

Optional:

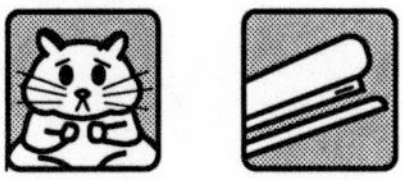

Hamster Stapler

How to Play:

First, you'll come up with your porn names based on the formula below. Then, you'll follow the instructions in the following steps to role-play a sexy porno!

Step One:

Come up with your porn names by using this formula:

First pet's name + the first street you lived on

Step Two:

Roll a die or randomly choose one card from the pile. Whatever number you get designates your porn title:

1/Ace: Passionate Pizza Delivery
2: Mile-High Hijinks
3: The Naughty Nerds
4: The Carnal Caveman
5: Camping Canoodles
6: The Handy Hottie

Step Three:

Write down the title and your porn names below to get started:

__________________starring ______________& ______________

Step Four:

Act out the scenes by rolling the die to find out what your next move will be! Keep playing until it gets too hot to handle!

1/Ace: Kiss anywhere
2: Touch anything
3: Caress anyplace
4: Massage anything
5: Fondle anywhere
6: Whisper your plans

"Free Pass" Lists

What you need:

Pencil

Optional:

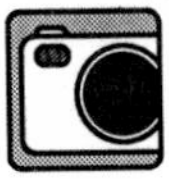

Camera

Tri-Pod

How to Play:
We all have our "celebrities-to-do" list. Let's turn the tables and see who your partner would pick for you. First, choose who will be player A and who will be player B. Using your designated section, complete the lists. Compare your answers in the end with what your partner actually says!

Player A:

Five celebrities whom you know your partner would want to do the nasty with:

1.
2.
3.
4.
5.

Five celebrities whom you would allow your partner one night with:

1.
2.
3.
4.
5.

Five celebrities whom you know your partner would never want to have sex with:

1.
2.
3.
4.
5.

Alright, now it's their turn...

"Free Pass" Lists

Player B:

Five celebrities whom you know your partner would want to do the nasty with:

1.
2.
3.
4.
5.

Five celebrities whom you would allow your partner one night with:

1.
2.
3.
4.
5.

Five celebrities whom you know your partner would never want to have sex with:

1.
2.
3.
4.
5.

Scoring:
Scoring? There's no win or lose here. The loss is that you're probably never going to be in a situation that'll allow you the opportunity to make love to any of the celebrities on your partner's "go for it" list. And if that opportunity ever came up, you'd better hope they listed some hottie and not five duds just to screw with you.

Whether you're watching TV or walking through the park, hold hands with your partner. Rev up the passion by gently rubbing their hand with your thumb or fingers.

I've Never...

What you need:

Pencil

Optional:

Beer Stein

How to Play:

Ever wonder about your partner's sexual history? Now's your chance to find out!

In this game, you'll need a player A and a player B. Player A goes first. Read the statements below to yourself and circle your answer: if you have done it or not, and if you think your partner has or hasn't done it. Then, player B will turn the page and answer their statements.

Scoring:

Afterward, read them aloud to each other and see if you guessed right, plus learn what your partner's answer was! You get a point for every correct answer. Tally your total points. The winner gets to plan your next romantic night out, and the loser has to clean the bathroom.

Player A:

I've never...joined the mile high club:

Have I done this:	no	yes
Do I think my partner has:	no	yes

I've never...done a striptease:

Have I done this:	no	yes
Do I think my partner has:	no	yes

I've never...had a one night stand:

Have I done this:	no	yes
Do I think my partner has:	no	yes

Player A cont.:

I've never...had a threesome:

Have I done this: no yes

Do I think my partner has: no yes

I've never...made out with someone of the same sex:

Have I done this: no yes

Do I think my partner has: no yes

I've never...done the deed in a public place:

Have I done this: no yes

Do I think my partner has: no yes

I've never...gotten caught in the act:

Have I done this: no yes

Do I think my partner has: no yes

I've never...had a fantasy about a teacher (or authority figure):

Have I done this: no yes

Do I think my partner has: no yes

I've never...done the walk of shame:

Have I done this: no yes

Do I think my partner has: no yes

Alright, now it's their turn...Player B, don't look at Player A's answers!

Player B:

I've never...joined the mile high club:

Have I done this:	no	yes
Do I think my partner has:	no	yes

I've never...done a striptease:

Have I done this:	no	yes
Do I think my partner has:	no	yes

I've never...had a one night stand:

Have I done this:	no	yes
Do I think my partner has:	no	yes

I've never...had a threesome:

Have I done this:	no	yes
Do I think my partner has:	no	yes

I've never...made out with someone of the same sex:

Have I done this:	no	yes
Do I think my partner has:	no	yes

I've never...done the deed in a public place:

Have I done this:	no	yes
Do I think my partner has:	no	yes

I've never...gotten caught in the act:

Have I done this:	no	yes
Do I think my partner has:	no	yes

I've never...had a fantasy about a teacher (or authority figure):

Have I done this:	no	yes
Do I think my partner has:	no	yes

I've never...done the walk of shame:

Have I done this:	no	yes
Do I think my partner has:	no	yes

I've Never...

Scoring:
So, once you're both done, read the statements aloud and tell each other what your answer would be, then compare those to what they thought you'd say! You get a point if you correctly guessed what they would have answered.

Tie-Breaker:
Seriously? You want me to come up with a tie-breaker? I just came up with all the other rules to this game. Fine...in the event of a tie, both of you have 5 minutes to come up with the dirtiest, raunchiest, most insanely ridiculous "I've Never" statement to stump your partner. The person who hasn't done that deed, wins! And if you both tie on this round, well then, you're just a couple of crazy sex maniacs and you deserve your own reality show.

Tally your results:

Player A: ____________

Player B: ____________

And the winner is:

____!

Congratu-freakin-lations. What's your reward for winning? Well, you get to pick what you want the loser's "punishment" to be! Laundry for a month? Some freaky sex act you've been wanting to try? It's all up to you, big kahuna.

"Sext" your partner throughout the day. Include why you love them, how they turn you on, what you have planned for the next night in...use your imagination.

What's the Definition?

What you need:

Paper

Pencil

Optional:

A Bucket of Sand

Spork

How to Play:
Out of the four definitions under each of these words or phrases, one is real. You have to figure out which one that is! Grab a pencil and some paper, and jot down your guesses as you go. Then, flip to page 99 for the answers and to see who won! The winner gets the title of Pervert King (or Queen). Congratulations, Your Pervertedness.

1. Donkey Punch
   a. kicking your legs behind you to hit a person or object
   b. punching a woman in the back of the head during sex
   c. a cocktail made with gin, vodka, and apple & pear juices
   d. an aphrodisiac made from a cocktail of donkey semen and cactus juice; popular in Uganda

2. Pabbed
   a. getting someone's pubes thrown in your face
   b. the Spanish word for "Bookshelf"
   c. slang for having had a marathon sex session
   d. when someone drew on your face because you passed out at the party the night before

3. Cack
   a. the slang term for a bent penis
   b. a baking utensil used to squeeze frosting onto a cake
   c. the word "Cock", said with a Boston accent
   d. the slimy coating that a snail trails behind itself

4. Prepuce
   a. the medical term for foreskin

b. the medical term for female vaginal fluid
c. the topmost point of a mountain
d. the sticky sap on a pine cone

5. Angina

a. a skin flap that develops inside the vaginal wall
b. a medical condition which involves suffocating and having painful spasms, like during a heart attack
c. a baby albatross
d. a disease that restricts a person's ability to stand on their tiptoes

6. Vajazzle

a. to give the female genitals a sparkly makeover with crystals to enhance their appearance
b. a small town in the Northern Great Plain region of Hungary
c. a theater-based dance performance influenced by 1960's Jazz
d. to shout "Jazz Hands!" and do the jazz hand motion during male ejaculation

7. Coccyx

a. the medical term for tailbone
b. a sex toy that wraps around the base of the penis to stimulate arousal
c. the medical term for eardrum
d. a cyst formed at the base of the penis

8. Fallacious

a. a person who enjoys giving oral pleasure to men
b. a sarcastic remark
c. a false statement
d. the act of a person being conniving or sneaky

9. Philatelist

a. a person who collects stamps
b. a list of people you wish to give oral sex to
c. the removable ring on a soda can
d. a religious philosopher

10. Cunning Linguist

a. an activist for abstinence-only sex education
b. a person who can speak multiple languages
c. someone who enjoys giving oral pleasure to women
d. a name given to 18th century poets in Great Britain

11. Cooter

a. a fishing lure that spins
b. the slang term for vagina
c. a species of turtle
d. a baby raccoon

12. Punanai

a. a small town in Sri Lanka
b. hawaiian slang for vagina
c. a pita wrap containing only vegetables
d. the peach fuzz that surrounds the belly-button

13. Trib

a. a person who is readily fluent; though often thoughtlessly, superficially, or insincerely so
b. the act of sucking a person's fingers seductively
c. the spring in a ball-point pen
d. a lesbian practice where two women rub their vaginas together during sex

14. Weenus

a. a breast-flavored pacifier used to wean children from breastfeeding
b. a common medical term for a very small penis
c. the skin on your elbows
d. the middle segment of an insect, between the head and thorax

15. Thrap

a. the bumpy texture on the edge of a quarter
b. a slang term for the act of masturbating
c. the heel strap on a pair of sandals
d. a soft tapping on the underside of the penis, used for sexual stimulation

Blind Bandit

What you need:

Blindfold

Pencil

Optional:

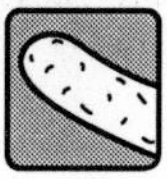

Cucumber

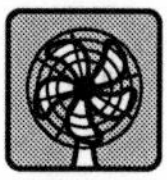

Fan

How to Play:

Two players, one blindfold. Start by each naming your one wager. The person who can say Honky Tonk Badonka Donk the fastest gets to wager first. You make these wagers up, but if you want me to do it for you, one of you says "If I win, you owe me dinner out" and one says "If I win, you give me a massage".

Once the wagers are placed, blindfold the contestant (the person who wagered last). The other person makes sure the contestant can't see, then proceeds to rub a random body part against them. The contestant has three chances to guess what they're feeling. If they guess correctly, they win. If not, they lose (obviously).

Switch roles. Play to the best of three rounds.

Wager One: ____________________

Wager Two: ____________________

Winner: ____________________

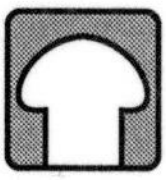

Plan an intimate night at home. Some ideas:
"Movie night" - buy some popcorn, rent a romantic movie and cuddle up together under a fluffy blanket.
"Tropical Getaway" - if you have access to a pool, lounge with your partner and soak up the rays, while drinking your favorite tropical beverage. At the end of the night, relax watching the sunset while enjoying tropical fruits, like mango, strawberries, and papaya.

Finish The Picture

What you need:

Pencil

Optional:

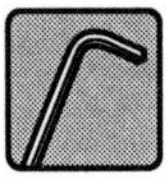

Allen Wrench

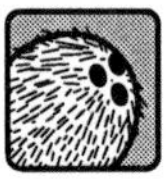

Coconut

How to Play:

On the next few pages are some sexy-looking squigllies, shapes and lines. Let's see if you can get your mind out of the gutter and finish the drawing in a non-raunchy way!

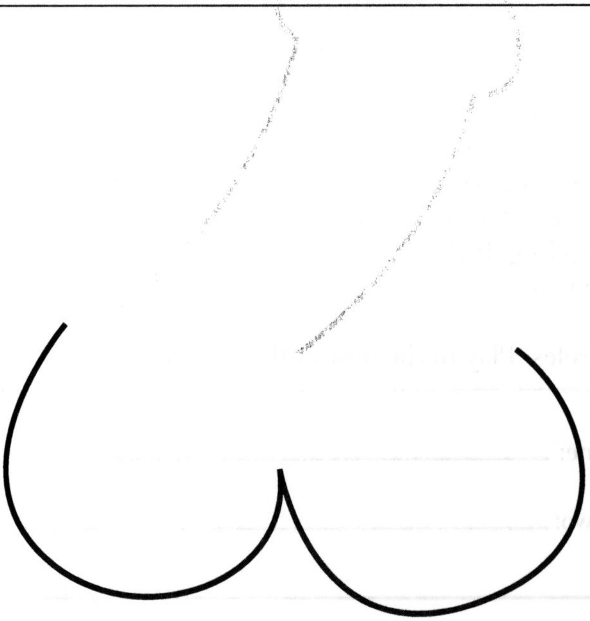

Finish The Picture

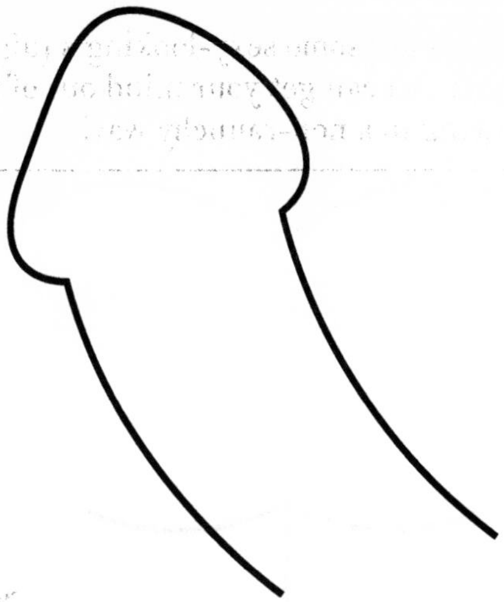

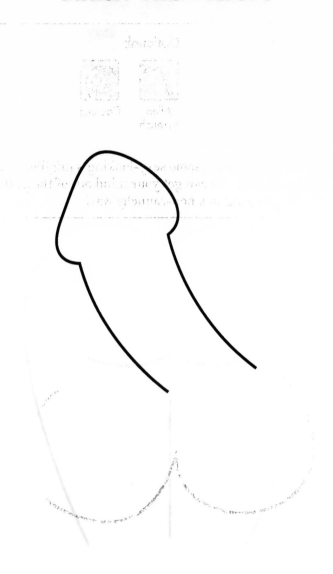

Finish The Picture

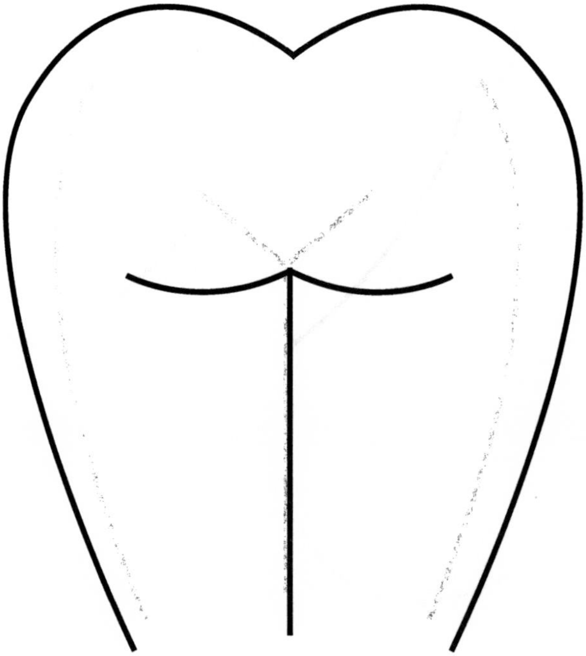

Finish The Picture

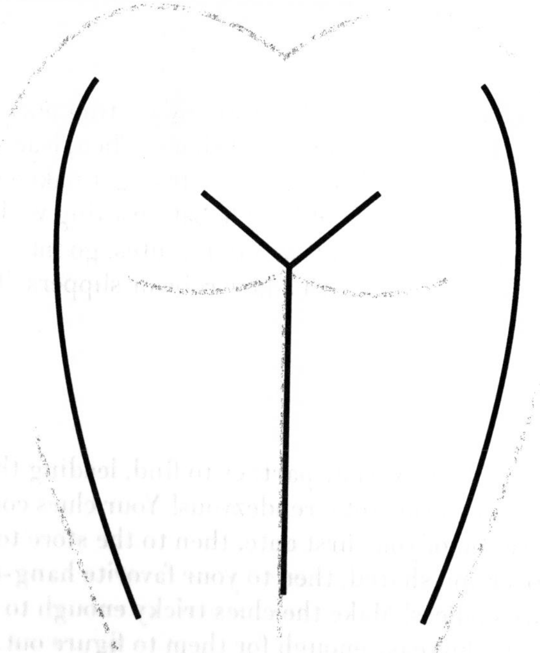

Sexy Scavenger Hunt

What you need:

Paper

Pencil

Optional:

Ham Sandwich

How to Play:

Use the ideas below to create sexy scavenger hunts for you and your partner that will get you both revved up during the day, resulting in a sexually explosive evening!

All About Them

Give your partner a relaxing night. Start by writing notes that instruct them to take off their coat and shoes. Then, lead them to the bathroom, all the while instructing to take get naked along the way. In the bathroom, have a hot bubble bath waiting with candles and relaxing music. After about twenty minutes, go into the bathroom and present them with a new robe or slippers. Then give them a full body massage.

Find the Clues

Create a game of clues for your partner to find, leading them on a chase that ends in a romantic rendezvous! Your clues could lead them to the location of your first date, then to the store to buy the first wine or beer you shared, then to your favorite hang-out...the possibilities are endless! Make the clues tricky enough to keep your partner guessing, but easy enough for them to figure out. In the end, lead them to the spot where you are waiting, ready to give the night some passion!

Happy Ending

Place a note near the door for your partner to find when they get home from work. Lead them to another note, then another. Each note should grow more and more sexual in nature. At the end, lead them to you, lying naked on the bed. Then, let the fun begin!

Teamwork

Below is a list of items that you two need to go find or buy together to have a steamy night! Copy them onto a sheet of paper, and head out to find them (create some of your own ideas as well!) When you get home, have a romantic, sensual night alone.

- A sensual movie
- Massage oil/lotion
- Alcoholic drink of choice
- Chocolate-dipped strawberries
- Music to put you in the mood
- Red lightbulbs
- Sexy panties/sexy boxers
- A sex toy/game
- Some type of lubricant

On Your Own

Similar to the game above, you both have to go out and find or buy the items listed below. The difference is that this time, you're on your own! Each of you copy the list and see who can find the most objects within a certain period of time (for example, three hours). It's fun trying to find them, and intriguing to think of what your partner might come home with!

- Some type of lubricant
- A sexy outfit for your partner to wear
- A sex toy/game
- Your partner's favorite sensual food/dessert
- Your partner's favorite alcoholic beverage
- A scented candle
- Some type of massage oil/lotion
- Some type of sensual music
- Something to tie your partner up with
- Something to tickle your partner with
- Something to tease your partner with

Sex Libs

What you need:

Pencil

Optional:

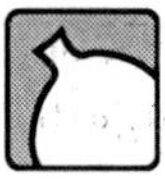

Whoopie Cushion

Screwdriver

How to Play:

One of you be the writer, and the other the player. You decide. The writer tells the player what words or phrases they need to fill in the blanks, then writes them in the spaces provided. Then, read the story aloud! Switch roles and play again.

"Stormy Shenanigans"

On a dark stormy night, I was sitting home alone enjoying a nice _____________ (Drink of Choice). As the rain tapped against the window, I began to think about _____________ (Significant Other). I started to think about being in _____________ (Travel Destination) together and it brought a smile to my face. While enjoying the delicious ___________ (Food) and thinking about seeing him/her wear his/her sexy ____________ (Article of Clothing), I started to get turned on.

As my mind turned to naughty thoughts, I felt the need to start rubbing my _____________ (Body Part)(s). Just then, I heard what sounded like a(n) _____________ (Animal) at the front door! It startled me so much that it almost made me _____________ (Verb). I was relieved to find out it was only _____________ (Significant Other).

I was so turned on, we immediately started _____________ (Verb Ending in "ing"). We gently started to massage each other's _____________ (Body Part)(s) with

our ____________(s). It wasn't long before we moved into the
Body Part

____________ and continued our fun.
Room of the House

We were in the middle of _______________ when all of a sudden
Verb Ending in "ing"

I felt a ____________ press against my ____________. I shouted
Noun — Body Part

"____________!" We both stopped for a moment and started to
Exclamation

____________. I was shocked at first, but then I thought adding a
Verb

_________________ to the mix would be fun as well.
Food

The passion was intense. I leaned in and whispered

"____________________________". The sweat was dripping off
Favorite Movie Quote

both our ______________(s). As we reached climax, I began to
Body Part

sing "_________________________" at the top of my lungs!
Favorite Song

We were both exhausted from all the ___________________ and
Verb Ending in "ing"

decided to go out for some ____________. It will forever go down
Food

as one of the most passionate nights I've ever experienced.

> The next time your partner is in the middle of their daily routine (doing their makeup, eating breakfast, etc.), surprise them by gently placing your hand on the small of their back, their shoulder, or their arm. Give them a small kiss somewhere, just to show how much you love them.

Sex Libs

"On the Set of a Porn Movie"

It had been 10 hours on the set of Raunchy ________________
Occupation Starting With "R"
________ and things were just not going well at all. Adult
Number
actors, Nine-__________ ______________ and __________
Unit of Measure Male First Name Adjective
__________ ________________ were both sick with
Body Part Female First Name
______________, so I had to stand in with ________________
A Disease Significant Other
to take their places.

We were so ___________ about ______________ in front of the
Emotion Verb Ending in "ing"
camera, since neither of us had tried anything like this before. But
we decided to take the __________ by the ______________ and
Animal Body Part - Plural
just go for it! To get in the mood, we gently ___________ each
Verb - Past Tense
other with a _______________.
Part of a Bird

Once we got good and _____________, we were ready to bite the
Adjective
____________. I lubed up my ________ with plenty of _________
Noun Body Part Liquid
and began to ___________ my partner _____________-style.
Verb Animal
Things were heating up, and we were _____________ with such
Verb Ending in "ing"
intensity, the ____________ slipped out, throwing me off my
Cylindrical Object
rhythm. I only had to think about _________ to get me back in the
Celebrity
mood and finish the job.

As we finished, the director yelled, "____________!", and we could
Exclamation
tell he was ____________ with our performance by the ________
Emotion Noun
on his face. The film made _____ dollars in the first month, which
Number
led us to the decision to continue in the porn industry as a career.

What's Your Sex IQ?

What you need:

Paper

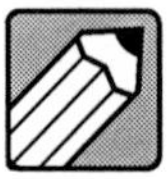

Pencil

Optional:

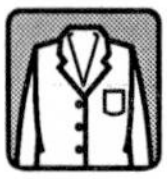

Lab Coat

How to Play:

Do you guys know anything about sex, or are you clueless like me? Take this short quiz together, then check out the answers on page 99 to tally your score to find out your sex IQ!

1. Is it possible for men to have multiple orgasms?
   a. Yes   b. No way

2. Who daydreams more while getting it on?
   a. Men   b. Women

3. You know what they say about big feet...
   True   False

4. Intercourse burns as many calories as running a mile
   True   False

5. Besides the bedroom, people most like to get it on in the:
   a. Car   b. Bathroom
   c. Backyard   d. Kitchen

6. How long does the average female orgasm last?
   a. Less than 5 seconds   b. 5-10 seconds
   c. 10-20 seconds   d. More than 20 seconds

7. How long does the average male orgasm last?
   a. Less than 5 seconds   b. 5-10 seconds
   c. 10-20 seconds   d. More than 20 seconds

8. In what season do more sexual activities occur?
   a. Winter   b. Summer

Scoring:

Go to page 99 to see what the answers are. Give yourself 20 points for each one you got right. Once you've tallied the points, check out the chart below to see where your sexual intelligence lies!

Below 70	Yikes. You probably shouldn't reproduce. But based on your knowledge of sex, you probably wouldn't know how anyways.
71-109	You're part of the average. You know enough to get by, but not enough to really "wow" somebody.
110+	You, my friend, are a sexual scholar. You could direct a porn movie.

Hide a little gift on the route you normally take for a walk with your sweetie. Direct your love to find the gift on your next walk.

Sexting

What you need:

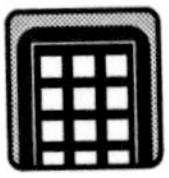

Cell Phone

Optional:

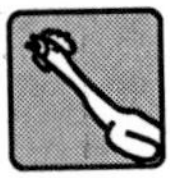

Rubber Chicken

How to Play:
Pick a day where you know the two of you will be apart from each other most of the day (ex; at work*). Throughout the day, "sext" each other on the hour, every hour. Be creative, and see what happens when you get home. To help get you started, I've given some suggestions below:

I was just thinking about "that thing" you did "that time"...

You drive me crazy when you (sexiest thing they do)...

I would love to try (insert sexy act here) with you!

Leave work ½ hour early today and I'll (fill in the blank) you when you get home!

I am shopping for a toy right now - any suggestions?

Let's get the kids into bed early tonight; I have something to show you!

Just thinking about taste-testing different areas of your body...

*Be responsible- I can't be held accountable if you get fired.

Pass the Ice Cube

What you need:

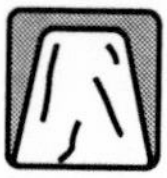
Ice Cube

Towel

Optional:

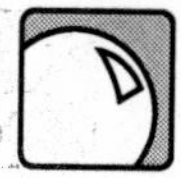
Ping Pong Ball

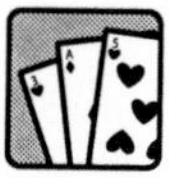
Cards

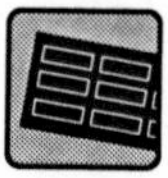
Chocolate

How to Play:

Decide who is going to be first. Grab an ice cube, put it in your mouth, then pass it to your partner by mouth. Keep passing it back and forth until it melts. Whoever has it when it completely melts loses!

Wanna make it more fun? Try some of these variations:

- Use a piece of chocolate or other fast-melting candy.
- Invite some friends!
- Use a playing card (suck and blow style).
- Use a ping pong ball (also, suck and blow style).

Scoring:

Here are some rewards for the person who wins, and some consequences for the person who lost. The more games you play, the better your chances of winning are!

Rewards:

You get a night out on the town, complete with dinner at your favorite restaurant, a movie or game (like putt-putt), plus a happy ending when you get home!

You get one day to relax and do nothing. Kick your feet up and watch TV, play games or just sleep!

Consequences:

You have to clean the entire home, apartment, or wherever you dwell. Top to bottom, make sure it's a deep clean.

You have to do all the laundry for a week.

Coupons

What you need:

Scissors

Optional:

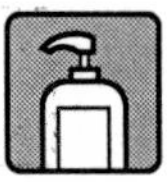

Lotion

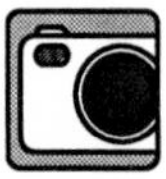

Camera

How to Play:

When you get presented with one of these coupons, you are required to do what's on them for your partner!

Good for one

Back Massage

Expires: Never

Good for one

Foot Massage

Expires: Never

Good for one

Striptease

Expires: Never

Truth or Dare

What you need:

Nothing

Optional:

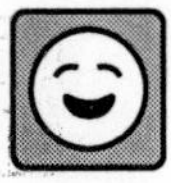

A Sense of Humor

How to Play:

Just like at slumber parties when you were a kid, this game is to coerce your partner into telling you a secret truth, or challenging them to do a raunchy dare! I've given you some examples below, but come up with your own to crank up the fun factor!

Tell me the truth...

- What TV show are you most embarrassed to watch?
- What feature are you most self conscious about?
- Have you ever flashed anyone?
- Have you ever had a one night stand?
- Have you ever given anyone a fake number?
- If you were the opposite sex for one day, what would you do?
- What is the kinkiest sex act you've done?
- Have you ever faked an orgasm?
- Who was your first crush?
- When was the last time you pleasured yourself?
- Have you ever masturbated anywhere inappropriate?
- What is your most perverted dream?
- Do you have any fetishes?

I dare you...

- To wear my underwear for the rest of this game
- To take a naked photo of yourself
- To reenact oral on my index finger
- To let me give you a bare bottom spanking
- To give me a back rub
- To down a drink
- To give me a lap dance
- To run naked through the house with the windows open

Places to Make Whoopie

What you need:

Dice Pencil

Optional:

56" TV Compass

How to Play:

This is a great game to play when things seem like they've gotten into a rut. Jot down twelve places where you and your partner would like to do the deed. Could be in your home, at some destination, or anywhere you haven't done it yet! Just don't put someplace where you'd get arrested.

Whenever you're in the mood, roll a pair of dice. Whatever number comes up is where you'll be getting it on! Have fun!

1. ______________________
2. ______________________
3. ______________________
4. ______________________
5. ______________________
6. ______________________
7. ______________________
8. ______________________
9. ______________________
10. ______________________
11. ______________________
12. ______________________

Massage Techniques

What you need:

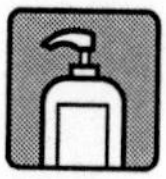

Lotion or Oil

Towel

Optional:

Blindfold

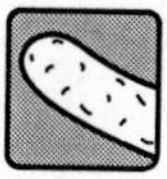

Cucumber

Lip Balm

How to Play:
Grab some oil or lotion, a towel and get into a comfy spot. Have fun using some of these massage techniques on each other.

Warning:
These are actual massage techniques, used by the pros, but I am not a chiropractor, doctor, or masseuse. And I'm not trying to give you health advice here. I seriously just did some research and put what I found in this book. So, please don't be a dummy when doing these or you could hurt someone.

Scalp Massage

The Set-up: The receiver lays on a bed or the floor, and the giver sits or stands behind their head.

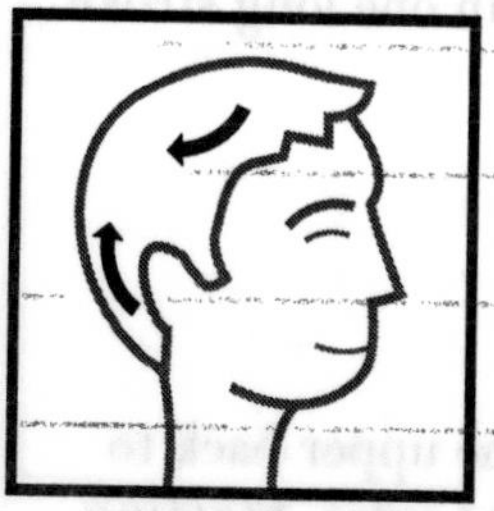

Step One:
It's best not to use oil for this massage, unless the receiver prefers it that way. Stroke your fingertips along the scalp from the forehead to the back of the head, then from the sides near the ears to the top of the head.

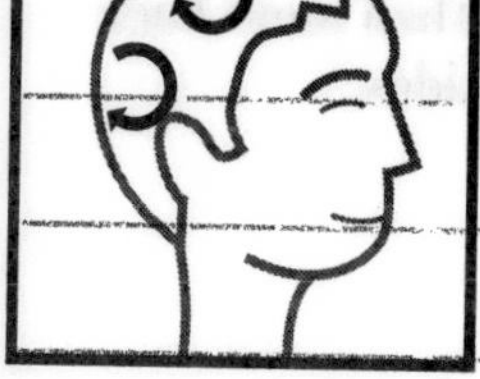

Step Two:
Brace your thumbs near the back of the head. Rotate your fingertips in small circles across the scalp from the front of the head to the back, extending down the neck a bit.

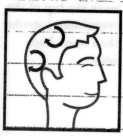

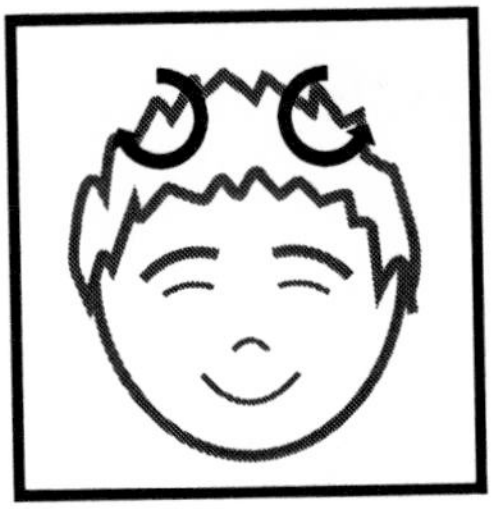

Step Three:
Then, massage in a circular pattern along the hairline, around the ears and across the back of the neck.

Shoulder & Back Massage

The Set-up: The receiver sits or lays in a comfy spot. The giver stands behind or straddles on top of the receiver's back.

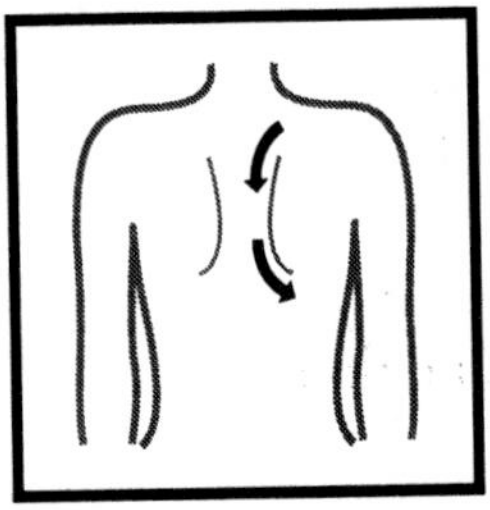

Step One:
Rub oil on your palms. Outline one shoulder blade with your fingers. Increase pressure by placing one hand on top of the other, then circle your palms around that shoulder blade. Repeat on the opposite side.

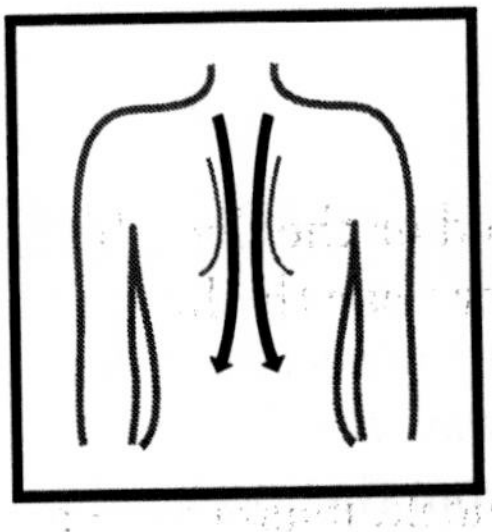

Step Two:
Place your palms on their back, fingertips pointing toward the lower back. Slowly glide your palms down the back in one long stroke.

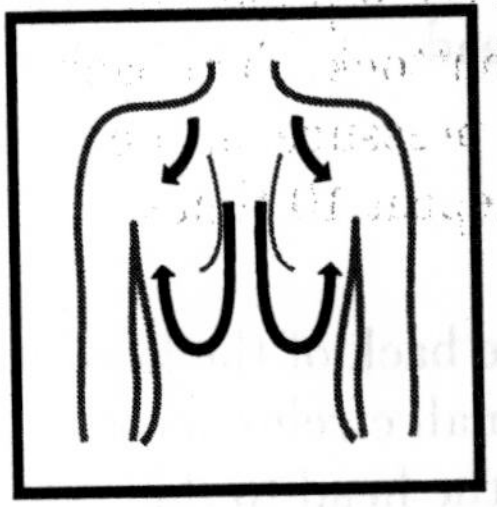

Step Three:
Make small strokes from the upper back to the lower, from center to the sides. Starting from the middle of the back near the top of the shoulder blades, move in one continuous stroke to the bottom of the blades, then move back upwards towards the outer sides.

Finger Massage

The Set-Up: This works if the receiver is either lying or sitting. The giver should be in a position that is comfortable for them to hold the receiver's hand.

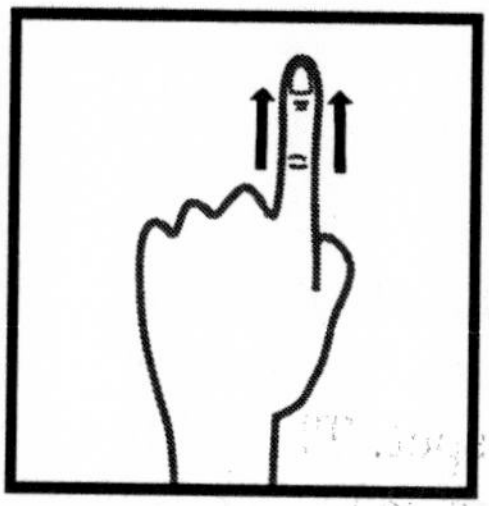

Step One:
Apply a small amount of oil or lotion to the receiver's hand. Wrap your fingers around their thumb. Squeeze three times, then gently stretch the thumb away from the palm. Repeat on the four fingers. (Make sure you avoid popping the joints by pulling too hard).

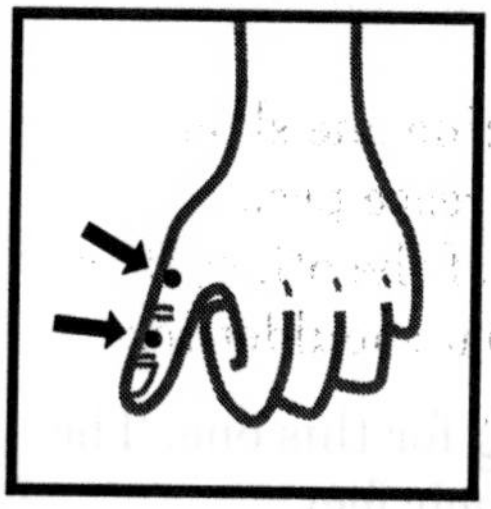

Step Two:
Then, starting back at the base of their thumb, press and release until you have pressed all the points from the base to the nail bed. At the nail bed, apply extra pressure, then slide off the tip of the thumb. Repeat on the four fingers.

Hips & Butt Massage

The Set-Up: The receiver lays face-down on a bed or the floor. The giver stands next to the bed or kneels on the floor near the hips.

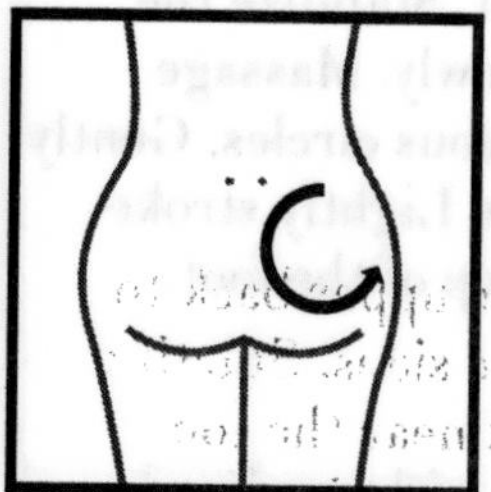

Step One:
Starting with the nearest cheek, massage in a broad, circular stroke from the hip joint to the upper buttock, then lower buttock, then back to the hip joint. Emphasize pressure on the stroke toward the center. Repeat 10 times.

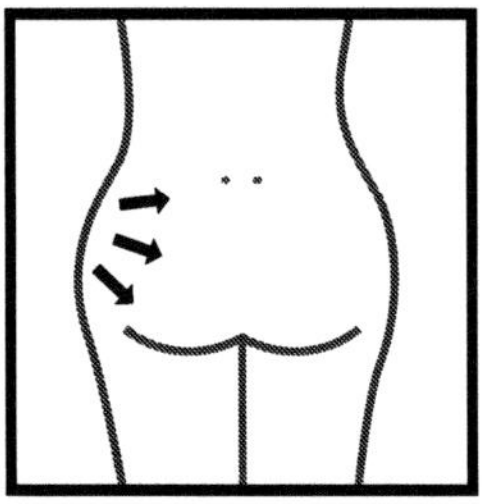

Step Two:
Then, massage in short, straight strokes 5 times as follows: from the hip joint toward the middle buttock, from the hip joint toward the lower buttock.

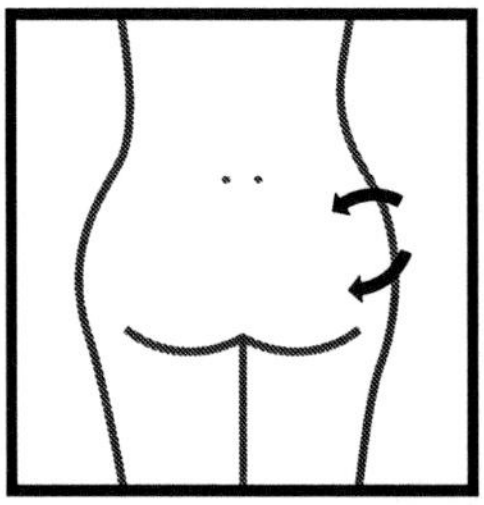

Step Three:
Reach across the receiver and place your hands on the opposite hip, near the bed or floor. Stroke your open palms from the hip to buttock. Alternate palms in a continuous flow, one after the other. Repeat the entire process on the other side.

Foot Massage

The Set-Up: The receiver can be sitting or lying for this one. The giver should stand or sit, facing the bottom of their feet.

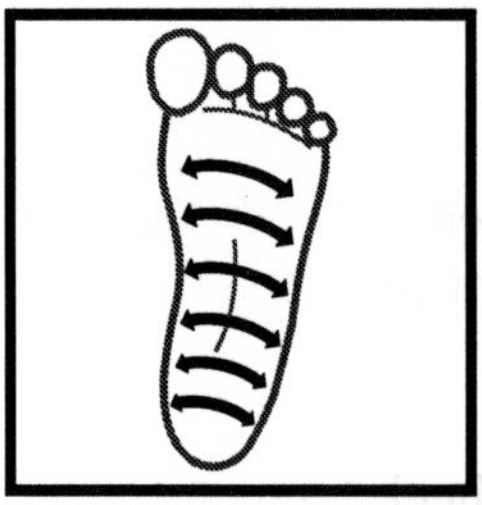

Step One:
(Note: Do not massage directly on the bones). Apply oil to both feet, but start with one foot at a time. Wrap your hand around the foot, squeeze, and slide from the ball to the outside of the foot, from ball to heel. Stabilize the ankle and rotate the foot slowly. Massage around the ankle in continuous circles. Gently squeeze, then pull, each toe. Lightly stroke between the bones on the top of the foot.

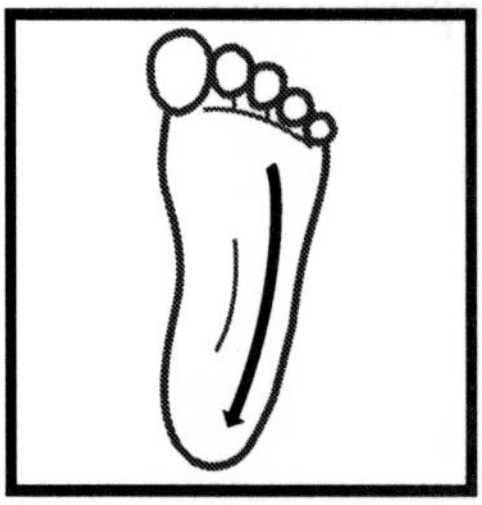

Step Two:
Support the top of the foot with one hand, and make a fist with the other. Slide your fist down the sole from below the toes to the heel. Lightly stroke the foot from ankle to toes. Repeat on the other foot.

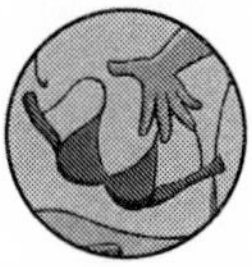

The Act

The Act. The Deed. The Nasty. Sex.

They all mean the same awesome, amazing, beautiful thing.

Hopefully playing this section will cause you and your partner to indulge in some form of the action listed above. If not, you're obviously not doing things right.

[illegible]

The contestant then guesses letters, but [illegible] guess wrong, they have to take off a piece of clothing from the list, starting at one. They can try to guess the phrase at any time. If they're right, they win!

If the contestant really sucks at this game and is stuck before the phrase is complete, they have one chance to guess the phrase. If they guess wrong, they have to do a nude-dance for the host to the tune of a song that the winner picks. If they guess right, they technically win, but they're still naked.

After the first game is done, players swap roles and play the next game.

Strip HungMan

What you need:

Pencil

Optional:

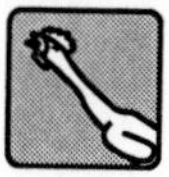

Rubber Chicken

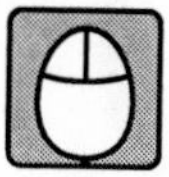

Computer Mouse

How to Play:

It's the same game as hangman, but with a twist: the person guessing has to strip if they get an answer wrong!

Start by picking who will be the host. Do this by competing in a good ol' fashioned draw. Stand back to back in the middle of a long room or hallway. Walk ten paces (that's long steps) away from each other. Once in place, one of you count to three out loud. On three, the first person to turn around to face the opponent, point their finger at them, and shout BANG! gets to be the host. The other person becomes the contestant.

Okay, so the host begins by writing down which items of clothing they want the contestant to take off, and in what order. Then, come up with a naughty phrase based on the theme I've provided. Tell the contestant how many letters are in the phrase and what the theme is.

The contestant then guesses letter by letter. Every time they guess wrong, they have to take off a piece of clothing from the list, starting at one. They can try to guess the phrase at any time. If they're right, they win!

If the contestant really sucks at this game and is nude before the phrase is complete, they have one chance to guess the phrase. If they guess wrong, they have to do a nudie-dance for the host to the tune of a song that the winner picks. If they guess right, they technically win, but they're still naked.

After the first game is done, players swap roles and play the next game.

Theme: A Sexual Fantasy

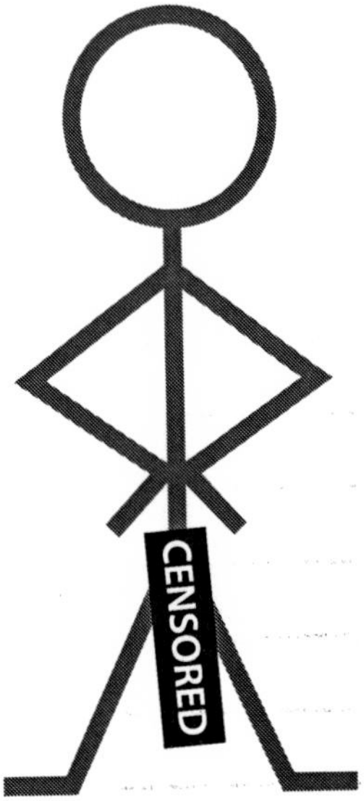

Take off:

1. ____________________
2. ____________________
3. ____________________
4. ____________________
5. ____________________
6. ____________________
7. ____________________
8. ____________________
9. ____________________
10. ____________________

Game play area:

A	B	C	D	E	F	G	H	I
J	K	L	M	N	O	P	Q	R
S	T	U	V	W	X	Y	Z	

Theme: A Funny Porn Title

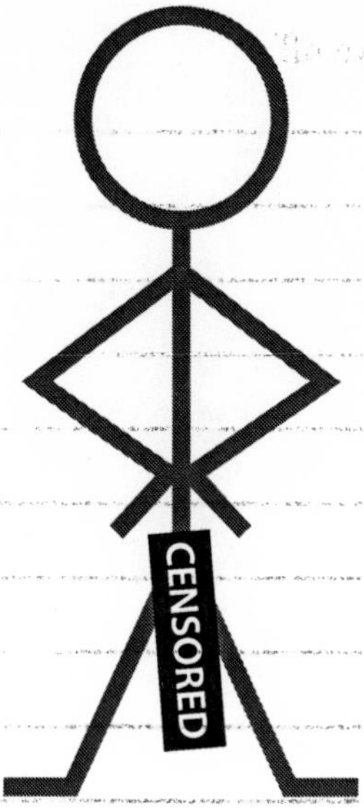

Take off:

1. ______
2. ______
3. ______
4. ______
5. ______
6. ______
7. ______
8. ______
9. ______
10. ______

Game play area:

A	B	C	D	E	F	G	H	I
J	K	L	M	N	O	P	Q	R
S	T	U	V	W	X	Y	Z	

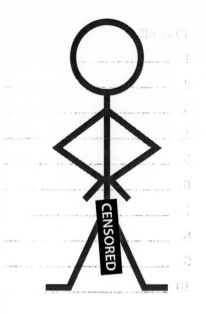

Theme: A Sexual Position

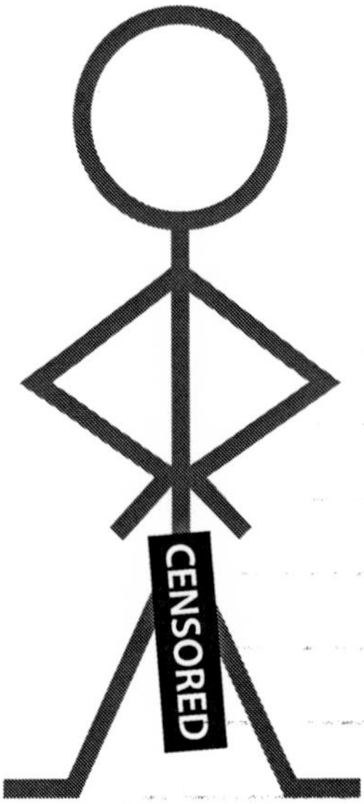

Take off:

1. ____________________
2. ____________________
3. ____________________
4. ____________________
5. ____________________
6. ____________________
7. ____________________
8. ____________________
9. ____________________
10. ____________________

Game play area:

A	B	C	D	E	F	G	H	I
J	K	L	M	N	O	P	Q	R
S	T	U	V	W	X	Y	Z	

Theme: A Sexual Euphemism

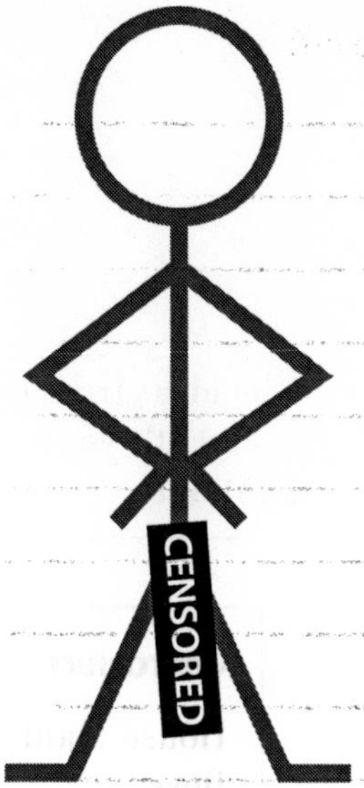

Take off:

1. ____________________
2. ____________________
3. ____________________
4. ____________________
5. ____________________
6. ____________________
7. ____________________
8. ____________________
9. ____________________
10. ____________________

Game play area:

A	B	C	D	E	F	G	H	I
J	K	L	M	N	O	P	Q	R
S	T	U	V	W	X	Y	Z	

You're the Author

What you need:

Pencil

Optional:

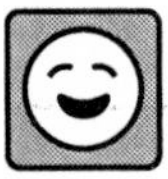

Sense of Humor

How to Play:
Write out a sexy story using at least one of the ideas from each category below. Mix and match them all you like; it's your story! Maybe have some fun afterward acting it out!

Genre	Settings	Characters
Horror	High-Rise	House Maid
Romance	Cabin	Boss
Comedy	Airplane	Pizza Guy/Gal
Drama	Office	Masseuse
Sci-Fi	Restaurant	Sugar Daddy
Indie	Vehicle	Cougar
Adventure	Boat	Girl Next Door
Fantasy	Fitting Room	Trainer
Crime Drama	Mansion	Doctor

Objects	Positions	Clothing
Vibrator	Missionary	Edible Undies
Cucumber	Doggie Style	Satin Boxers
Cantaloupe	Couch Canoodle	Silk Robe
Sex Swing	Hang Ten	Lacy Bra
Hot Tub	Lusty Leg Lift	Black Panties
Mirrors	Love Triangle	Fishnets
Video Camera	Sexy Sprinkler	Stilettos
Camera	Erotic End	Cowboy Hat
Shower	Sensual Spoon	Leather Catsuit

by

Sexy M.A.S.H.

What you need:

Pencil

Optional:

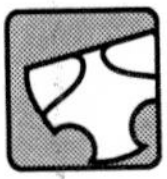

Diaper

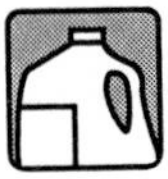

5 Gallons of Milk

How to Play:
First, decide who will be the writer by seeing who has the longer middle finger (on your right hand). Then, the writer will use the chart on the next page to begin. The player gets to decide what goes in each category, and the writer writes it down. Duh.

Scoring:
Once all the categories are complete, the writer and the player will do different things at the same time. Pay attention. The player will begin counting in their head, while the writer begins drawing small dash marks in the "Dash Area" at the bottom of the game page. When the player decides enough is enough, they will say "Nana Nana Boo Boo" to indicate that they want the writer to stop drawing. Or they can just say "Stop", whatever works.

The writer then counts up how many dashes they drew.

Using that number and starting with the letter M, the writer counts the number of dashes while moving from answer to answer. When they reach the number, they'll cross out that answer. For example, if the number is four, they'll do this: M, A, S, H, then cross out H. When you only have one answer in each category, including the word MASH, the game is complete. In case you didn't know, M.A.S.H. stands for Mansion, Apartment, Shack and House.

The writer will then write the answers below the game form, then read them aloud to the player. Switch roles and play again!

M A S H

Who you do the deed with	What room you do it in
1.	1.
2.	2.
3.	3.
4.	4.
What you do it on	**What object/toy you use**
1.	1.
2.	2.
3.	3.
4.	4.
How it's done (position)	**What you do afterwards**
1.	1.
2.	2.
3.	3.
4.	4.

Where you do the deed (MASH): ______________________

Who you do the deed with: ______________________

What room you do it in: ______________________

What you do it on: ______________________

What object/toy you use: ______________________

How it's done: ______________________

What you do afterwards: ______________________

Dash Area

M A S H	
Who you do the deed with 1. 2. 3. 4.	What room you do it in 1. 2. 3. 4.
What you do it on 1. 2. 3. 4.	What object/toy you use 1. 2. 3. 4.
How it's done (position) 1. 2. 3. 4.	What you do afterwards 1. 2. 3. 4.

Where you do the deed (MASH): ______________________

Who you do the deed with: ______________________

What room you do it in: ______________________

What you do it on: ______________________

What object/toy you use: ______________________

How it's done: ______________________

What you do afterwards: ______________________

Dash Area

Best Sexy Superpower

What you need:

Pencil

Optional:

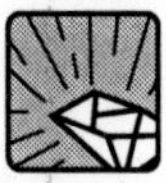

Kryptonite

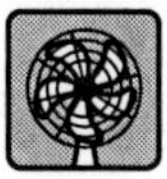

Fan

How to Play:

We all agree that the x-ray vision would be a sexy, albeit creepy, superpower. What about some other powers that could be super-sexy? Invisibility? Mind-control? Figure out what would be your favorite superpower to woo someone and compare it to your partner's choice! If you feel like it, draw your superhero character below. Or, make it more interesting and draw each other's character!

Wrestling Move or Sex Act?

What you need:

Pencil

Optional:

Wrapping Paper

How to Play:

On the next page are twenty phrases. Fourteen of them are wrestling moves, while six of them refer to acts of sexual pleasure. You have to guess which are the sex acts.

Choose who will be player 1 and who will be player 2, then list your guesses in the appropriate columns below the words.

Once you're done, go to page 99 for the answers! (No peeking! If you do, you are a cheater, and therefore a pumpkin eater.)

Scoring:

I'm gonna change this up a bit. Instead of "whoever has the most right, wins", how about whoever guessed a sex act correctly gets to try that act with their partner, at a time of their choosing? You like that? Yeah, I thought you would.

Tie-breaker:

Grab a couple pieces of paper. You already have a pencil, so you're good there. Okay, whoever can draw the best rendition of the Spanish Inquisition wins. Go! Have no artistic ability, or have no clue what the hell happened during the Spanish Inquisition? Then whoever lost their virginity first wins.

Cooking together brings you closer, so plan an at-home dinner date with your favorite wine. Don't forget some romantic music and lots of playfulness as you cook!

the tight squeeze

the spider web

the flying lariat

the testicular claw

the head game

trapping headbutts

the battering ram

the shining wizard

stink face

face wash

the mounted elbow

the linguini

the pendulum

rolling thunder

the pinwheel

go to sleep

the butt drop

dragon whip

mover and shaker

Player 1: ______________________

____

____

____

____

____

Player 2: ______________________

____

____

____

____

____

Soooo, who won?? I can't handle it - the suspense is killing me!!

Not really.

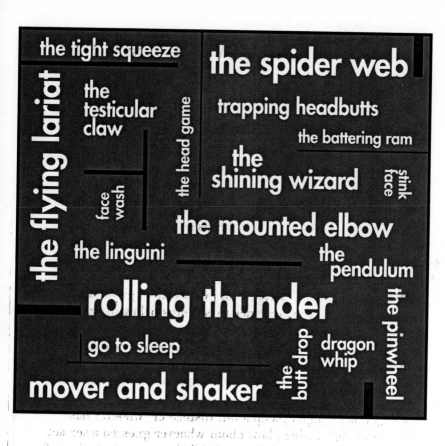

Sex Charades

What you need:

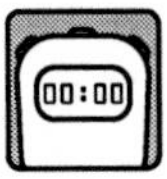

Stopwatch -or- Timer

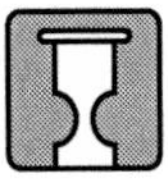

Optional:

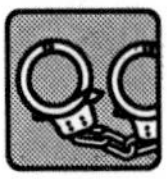

Handcuffs

Cattle Prod

How to Play:

On the next two pages, I've listed a variety of intimate and sexual actions. Each of you rip out one sheet, but try not to look at what's on your partner's page!

Decide who will go first, then set a timer for two minutes, or use a sand timer from another game. Come up with some of your own charades if you want to make the game a bit more interesting!

Act out the actions without speaking to see if they can guess what you're doing!

Scoring:

Tally who wins after each round. If they guessed what you acted out, they get a point. If they had no clue because you're that good of an actor (or that bad of one), you get one point.

At the end, whoever has the most points wins and gets to pick the next movie you guys go out to see.

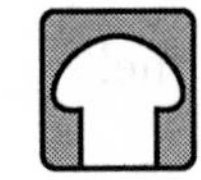

Lay out some blankets and pillows and have a picnic on the floor at home together!

Sex Charades - Player One

Multiple Orgasms
Booty Call
Walk of Shame
One Night Stand
Banana Hammock
Manscaping
Edible Underwear
Tantric Sex
(Write your own idea here)
(Write your own idea here)

Sex Charades - Player Two

Easy Access
Kegel Exercises
Hung like a Horse
Virgin
Quickie
The Morning After
Ménage a Trois
Foot Fetish
(Write your own idea here)
(Write your own idea here)

Toy Chest

What you need:

Pencil

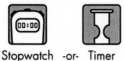

Stopwatch

-or-

Timer

Optional:

Frozen Hot Dog

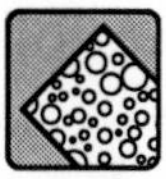
Sponge

How to Play:
Set a timer for three minutes, or use a sand timer from a board game. Get yourself into position with this book and a pencils, each of you using one of the next two pages for your drawings. Sit or lay across from each other. Spread the book open between the two of you, so that the spine is running horizontally between you and you each have one page to work on.

Start the timer, and draw all the objects that you think your partner would like to have in their personal sex "toy chest".

Scoring:
Once the time is up, drop your pencils! Compare your ideas to their reality. Then maybe go buy some of those things you wish they had.

Surprise your partner by role-playing their favorite fantasy when they least expect it.

Toy Chest

◄ Player A draws here ◄

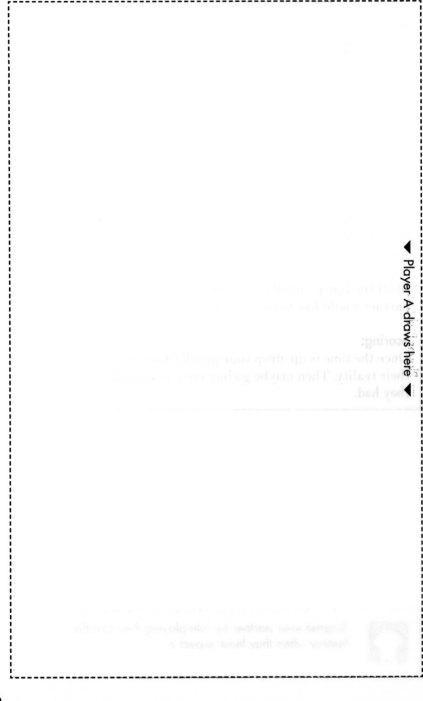

Toy Chest

▶ Player B draws here ▶

7 Minutes of Pleasure

What you need:

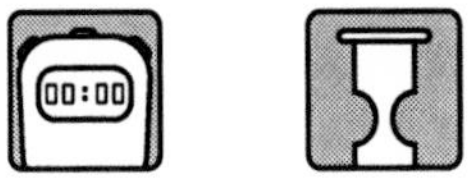

Stopwatch -or- Timer

Optional:

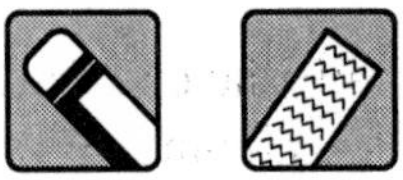

Lip Balm Gum

How to Play:

Grab a stopwatch or other timer, and set it to go off every minute for seven minutes. If you don't have an interval timer, just watch a clock. Or if you're really adventurous, ask a friend to observe and yell every time a minute is up. Whatever works for you.

Get naked and sit across from each other. For this game, we're going to refer to the younger person as player 1 and the older as player 2. Player 1 will go first. Why? Because I said so.

Every minute, you'll be changing it up. Start with minute one, obviously, then move on as indicated. Once your seven minutes is up, switch roles and keep going until you can't hold out any longer. Now go!

0:1 Sit behind your partner. Using only your hands, run your fingers through your partner's hair and gently massage their scalp.

0:2 Tell your partner to lie flat on their stomach. Using only your fingertips, start at the feet and gently brush your hands up our partner's body toward the head. Avoid touching any "private" areas.

0:3 Now, lightly move your fingers back towards their feet, again avoiding their "private" areas until you reach the bottoms of their feet.

0:4

Next, you'll gently start kissing their erogenous zones from feet to head: Feet, Back of Knees, Buttocks, Wrists, Nape of Neck, and Ears.

0:5

Then, tell Player 2 to turn onto their back. This time, gently kiss from top to bottom: Lips, Neck, Breasts/ Nipples, Stomach, Genitals and Inner Thighs.

0:6

Use your tongue, lips or hands to touch anywhere on their body, except those "private" areas.

0:7

Now, you'll have this last minute to focus on only the fun parts. Once the time is up...STOP!

Now switch roles and see how long you can last!

Next time you go out to dinner, pretend you're on a first date. Play footsies for at least ten minutes; look into each other's eyes; hold hands all night. Maybe you can even "run out of gas" on the ride home. ;-)

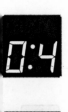

Hot Spots

What you need:

Pencil

Optional:

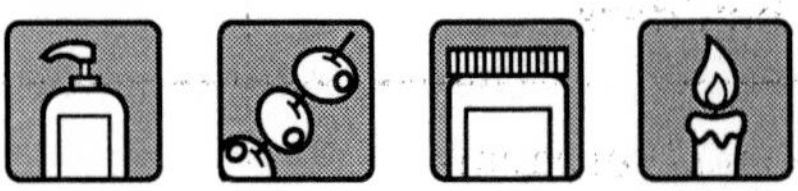

Lotion | Olives | Peanut Butter | Candles

How to Play:

This game will help you determine your partner's most sensitive areas - those pleasure spots that make them squirm (in a good way). Both of you get naked - NOW. (I've always wanted to say that).

Using your hands, feet, tongue, a feather, a vibrator, some hot wax, or whatever else you can think of depending on how adventurous you are, play around with the body parts listed below on your partner. Once you discover something they love, write it down on the chart and give it a rating from 1-10 (10 being the best). If you find something that makes them punch you in the head, you'd better make damn sure you remember not to do it again. There are some blank spots too, in case you get super-crazy and decide to explore other areas.

I've started you off with an example in the top row, just in case you really don't understand the simple instructions above.

Body Part:	What they like/hate:	Rating:
Inner Thigh	She loved when I slowly licked in the crease between her thigh and her "hoo-haa".	10
Scalp		
Ear Lobes		
Neck		

Body Part:	What they like/hate:	Rating:
Nape of Neck		
Shoulders		
Arms/Forearms		
Hands/Wrists		
Breasts/Nipples		
Stomach/Belly Button		
Hips		
Penis/Clitoris		
Testicles		
Inner Thighs		
Butt		
Back of Knees		
Feet		

Now switch roles to see what your partner enjoys.

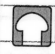

Gently massage your partner's ear while doing an everyday, menial task (like cleaning up after dinner).

Body Part:	What they like/hate:	Rating:
Scalp		
Ear Lobes		
Neck		
Nape of Neck		
Shoulders		
Arms/Forearms		
Hands/Wrists		
Breasts/Nipples		
Stomach/Belly Button		
Hips		
Penis/Clitoris		
Testicles		
Inner Thighs		
Butt		
Back of Knees		
Feet		

How Well Do You Know Your Partner in the Bedroom?

What you need:

Paper

Pencil

Optional:

Mullet Wig

How to Play:

What do you think your partner would say? Each of you grab a piece of paper and a pencil. Read each question aloud, then write down your answers. After you're done, compare how well you know each other!

1. How does your partner prefer sex initiation:
   a. randomly
   b. just let it happen
   c. schedule it
   d. never

2. Would your partner:
   a. turn the lights off
   b. leave the blinds open
   c. keep the lights on
   d. go under the covers

3. How long would your partner prefer foreplay to last?
   a. 5 min
   b. 10 min
   c. 20 min
   d. What's foreplay?

4. Do they prefer top or bottom? How about front or back?

5. What would they do afterwards?
   a. sleep
   b. eat
   c. smoke
   d. watch TV
   e. rev up for another round

6. Would they be open to using toys?
   a. yes
   b. no

7. Food in the bedroom: a complete turn-on or turn-off?

____

8. What does your partner think about during sex?
   - a. you
   - b. a celebrity
   - c. someone else they know
   - d. their household to-do list

9. How long does your partner think sex should last?
   - a. 5 min
   - b. 20 min
   - c. 45 min
   - d. An hour or more

10. What is your partner's role-playing fantasy?

____

11. If you two got caught making whoopie in a public place, your partner would:
    - a. be embarrassed, blush and take their punishment
    - b. proudly announce that they were "gettin' some"
    - c. run as fast as they can

12. Immediately after sex, your partner usually
    - a. falls asleep
    - b. gets something to eat
    - c. cuddles you
    - d. takes a shower

13. What would be your partner's favorite Kama Sutra position?
    - a. Now and Zen
    - b. Bucking Bronco
    - c. Yes, Yes, YES!
    - d. Supernova

14. How often would your partner like to have sex?
    - a. once a week
    - b. three times per week
    - c. daily
    - d. once a month
    - e. only during the blue moon

15. What type of porn video would your partner prefer?
    - a. Team Tantric: The Sporting Event with No Half-Time!
    - b. The Erotic Extra-Terrestrial: Learning Martian Moves
    - c. The Pulsing Pool Boy: He's Ready to Clean Your Drain
    - d. Mischievous Maids II: I'll Show You My Feather Duster

Do You Know Your Sex Stats?

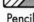

What you need:

Paper Pencil

Optional:

Ruler

How to Play:

Are you part of the norm when it comes to sex issues? Work together to answer these questions based on what you think, or know, about people's sexual activities. Answers are on page 99!

1. Do most people prefer the light on or off?
2. The average male loses his virginity at what age?
3. The average female loses her virginity at what age?
4. The number of times per year that the average person has sex is:
5. The number of minutes the average person spends on foreplay is:
6. What is the percentage of women who have faked an orgasm at least once in their life?
7. What is the average number of sex partners in a lifetime for men?
8. What is the average number of sex partners in a lifetime for women?
9. What is the average length of sexual intercourse in minutes?
10. The percentage of men who think about sex several times a day is:
11. The percentage of men who think about sex less than once per month is:
12. The percentage of women who want regular sex after four years of marriage is:

Source: Kinsey Report, National Center for Health Statistics. Date Verified: 3/27/2012

Would Your Partner...

What you need: | **Optional:**

Paper | Pencil | Beer Stein | Ham Sandwich

How to Play:
What do you think your partner would say? Grab a piece of paper and a pencil. Read each question aloud, then write down your answers. After you're done, compare how well you know each other!

- Would your partner try a sex swing? (Y/N)
- Would your partner try a threesome? (Y/N)
- Would your partner try swinging? (Y/N)
- Has your partner had a one night stand? (Y/N)
- If your partner could choose any toy to use in the bedroom, it'd be a ________.
- Would your partner would rather have a serious make-out session under a cabana on a beach during the sunset, or in front of the fireplace in a cozy cabin during a thunderstorm?
- Your partner's most erogenous zone is ___________.
- Your partner would say they are completely sexually satisfied. (Y/N)
- Your partner would like to have sex more often. (Y/N)
- Your partner would like to have sex less often. (Y/N)
- Your partner would say that, more often than not, you take charge in the bedroom. (Y/N)
- Your partner prefers to dominate over being dominated. (Y/N)

Versus

What you need:

Paper

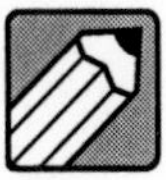
Pencil

Optional:

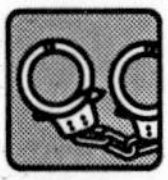
Handcuffs

How to Play:

How different are you two? How are you similar? Can we possibly start any "dating show on an island"-type drama between you with this game? I don't know...let's see!

Listed below are different options for things involving sex. You guys have to let each other know which you'd prefer, and why.

Tied Up vs. Blindfolded

Lights vs. Candles

Lingerie vs. Pajamas

Striptease vs. Lap Dance

Socks On vs. Socks Off

TOP vs. BOTTOM

Cuddling vs. Making me a Sammich

Whip Cream vs. Chocolate Syrup

MANUAL vs. BATTERY

whips vs. chains

Front Door vs. Back Door

Porn Movie vs. Porn Magazine

Bed vs. Couch

Guess the Length

What you need:

Pencil

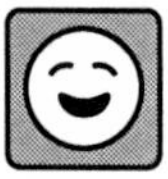

A Sense of Humor

Optional:

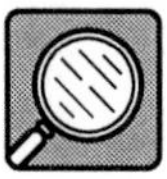

Magnifying Glass

How to Play:

Alrigh guys, time to face the music. Jump out of those skivvies and see how you "measure up". Just remember, it's not the size of the boat, but the motion of the ocean. Or so they say.

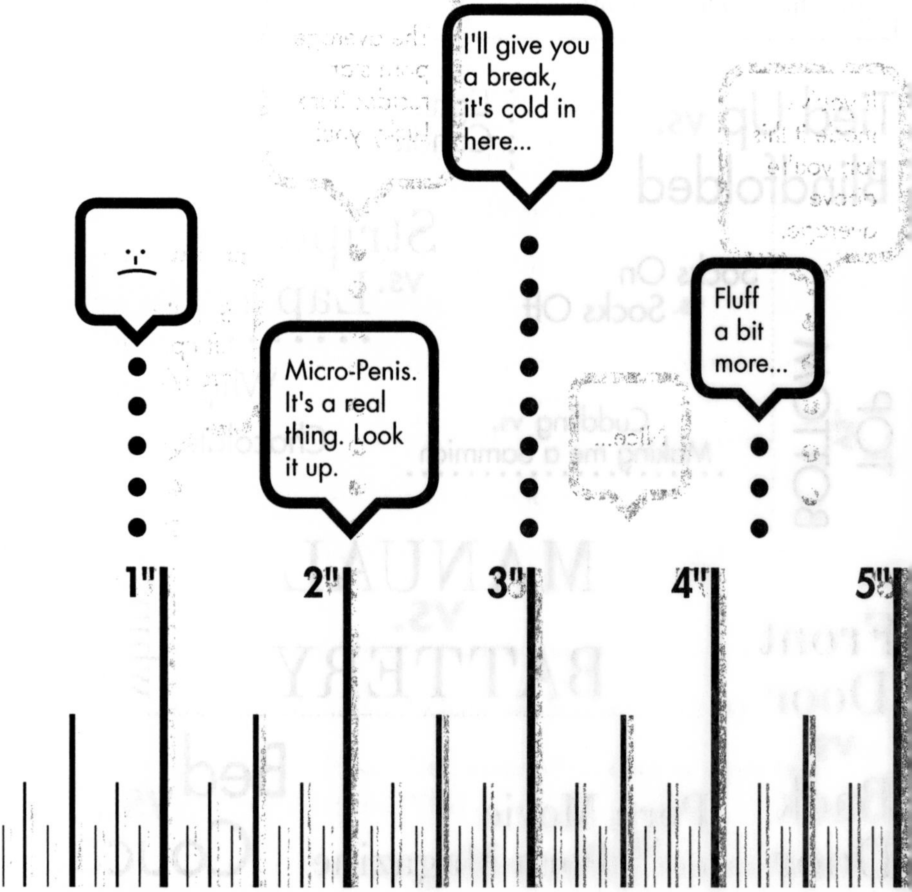

* These measurements are, in fact, true to scale. Add maybe 1/8" to compensate for the crease, but otherwise - no cheating!

Objects in crease are larger than they appear.

If you've made it this far, you're above average.

Nice...

The average porn star resides here. Lucky you!

Shut the eff up, you are lying.

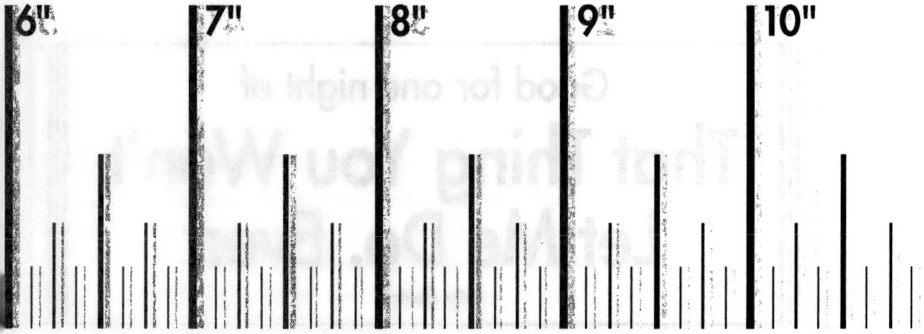

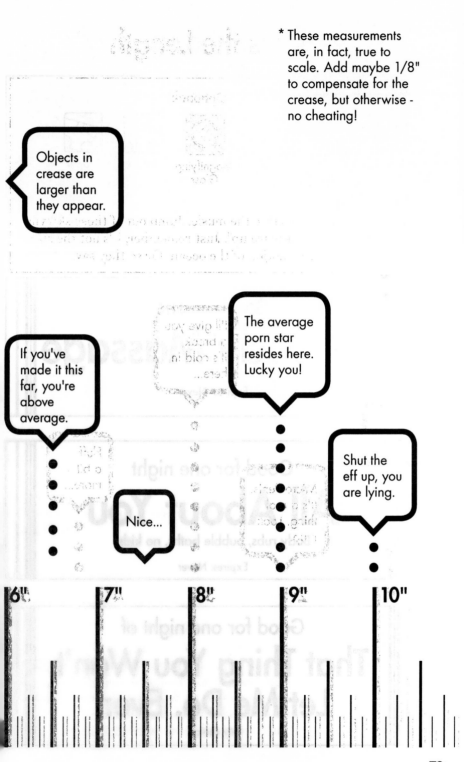

Coupons

What you need:

Scissors

Optional:

Towel

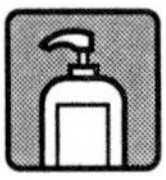

Lotion

Diaper

How to Play:
When you get presented with one of these coupons, you are required to do what's on them for your partner!

Good for one
Full Body Massage
Expires: Never

Good for one night
All About You
Body rubs, bubble baths, no kids.
Expires: Never

Good for one night of
That Thing You Won't Let Me Do. Ever.
My choice.

Double Dare

What you need:

Nothing

Optional:

56" TV

Glue

How to Play:

Similar to the previous "Truth or Dare" game on page 35, but I've upped the ante with new dares that'll have you blushing in no time. Come up with some of your own too!

I double dare you...

- To try a sex position of my choice
- To let me ice your nipples
- To let pour hot candle wax on you
- To let me lick/suck any part of your body I choose for 30 seconds
- To lick/suck any part of my body I choose for 30 seconds
- To masturbate in front of me for 30 seconds
- To act out your best fake orgasm
- To kiss my neck for 1 minute
- To give me oral sex for 1 minute
- To watch a porno with me
- To reenact a porn scene with me
- To do a striptease for me, lasting at least 5 min (or until I can't handle it!)

Leave your partner "Naughty Notes"; little sayings, thoughts or actions that they will find throughout the day reminding them of the passion they enjoy with you.
Example: I love how your booty sways when you walk!
Example: Later on, I'd like to lick your...

Use Your Senses

What you need:

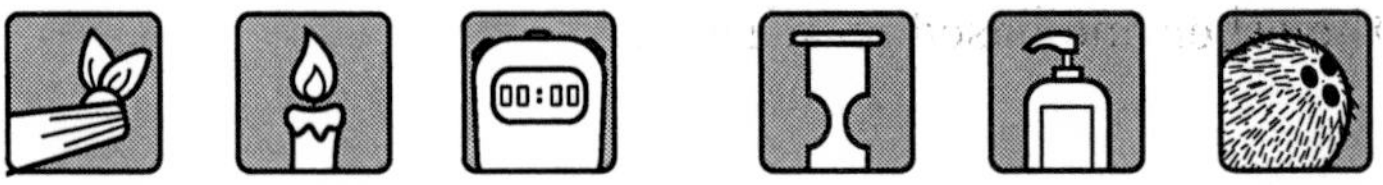

Blindfold Candle Stopwatch -or- Timer Lotion Some types of foods

How to Play:

Below are five games, each tailored to one of your senses. You can play these all consecutively, or on a whim.

Touch

- Set a timer for 20 minutes.
- Using a scarf or tie as blindfolds, "blind" you and your partner.
- Start the timer.
- Using only your sense of touch, find your partner's best pleasure zones and explore!

Taste

- Each of you find four items to "taste-test", but don't let your partner know what you've picked.
- One of you blindfold the other.
- Using only taste and smell, sensually make your partner guess what foods they are eating as you feed it to them.
- Once one of you is done, it's the other's turn!

Hearing

- Find the most comfortable spot in your home.
- Turn off all the lights in that room; and light some candles.
- Get into a comfy position next to your partner, so you're able to whisper in their ear.
- Giving yourself a time limit of three minutes, tell your partner what you'd like to do to them, and what you want them to do to you.
- The catch is, the person being spoken to cannot speak back!
- Once one partner is finished, it's the other's turn.

Sight

- Get as comfortably nude in front of each other as you can (if that means just wearing skimpy clothes, that's fine!)
- Set a timer for ten minutes.
- Every minute, trade off telling each other exactly what you love about the other one based on what you see.

Smell

- Either find, buy or borrow a variety of massage lotions/oils (two-four works great), but keep them a secret from your partner.
- Get your partner ready for a massage, but blindfold them.
- Using only their sense of smell, make them pick their favorite scent from the oils you got.
- Once they choose, give them a full-body rub down!

Toast each other when you sit down to dinner. It doesn't need to be over bubbly or wine; a glass of water or iced tea will do just as well. Tell each other something you love about them and then drink to it!

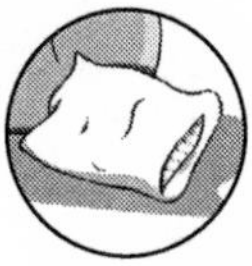

Afterglow

That moment when you're relaxed, content and satisfied (or so we hope).

Then your partner ruins it by telling you to go make them a sammich.

What's Your Excuse?

What you need:

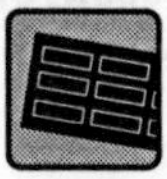

Chocolate

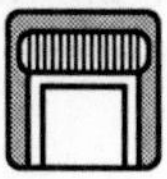

Ibuprofen

Optional:

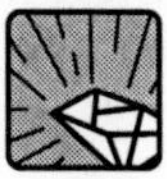

Kryptonite

How to Play:

Next time your partner gives you some lame excuse as to why they can't have sex, use these awesome (and factual) "sex benefits" to woo them into the sack!

If they say...	Then you say...
I have a headache.	**Sex will ease that pain!** Half of women report that sex actually eases headaches, says Randolph W. Evans, M.D., clinical prof of neurology at the Baylor College of Medicine in Houston.
Sex will get me too wound up.	**Oh no it won't...** Orgasms release endorphins that will put you to sleep faster than counting sheep.
I've got a cold.	**I'll be your antibiotic...** According to a study from Wilkes University in Wilkes-Barre, Pennsylvania, weekly sex contributes to about a 30 percent hike in immunoglobulin A, an antibody that fights infection.
I just don't have the sex drive.	**More is better.** One of the key hormones that fuels the sex drive is testosterone, which in turn, is produced when making love. In other words, the more you do it, the more you want it.

If they say...	Then you say...
I have heart problems.	**I have "heart"-ON problems...** Get the go-ahead from your doctor, first. However, humping lowers blood pressure, which can help reduce your chance of heart disease.
I'm busy and I don't have the energy to do it all.	**It'll increase your motivation!** Again, those endorphins - they can make you feel more motivated after a nice roll in the hay.
I feel fat.	**Let's work out!** A 30 minute hump-fest can burn up to 200 calories.
I don't feel like we are close anymore.	**Let's reconnect!** Sex can make you feel more connected to your partner, as it releases oxytocin.
I have cramps.	**Sex can fix that!** Sex is the remedy- contracting uterine and pelvic floor muscles during sex may reduce the pain.
I'm too tired.	**Let me wake you up.** Like during exercise, heavy breathing during sex sends oxygen to the brain and other vital organs, helping your body work more efficiently.
I'm too sore.	**Sex will make you feel less pain.** During orgasms, your pain threshold increases more than 100 percent, easing muscle and joint aches.

Do You Know Your Partner's Intimate Side?

What you need:

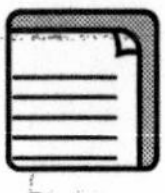
Paper

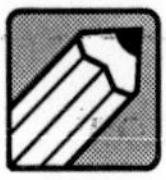
Pencil

Optional:

Allen Wrench

How to Play:

Using two separate pieces of paper, answer these questions from both yours and your partner's point of view. Afterward, share your answers with your partner to find out if you know them intimately, and learn something about them if you don't!

- Where is your partner most ticklish?
- Does your partner enjoy cuddling?
- Does your partner prefer holding hands, putting their arm around you, or having your arm put around them?
- What is the deepest thing your partner has ever shared with you?
- Where does your partner like to be massaged?
- Does your partner enjoy making future plans with you?
- What is their biggest life goal?
- How does your partner express their love?
- What intimate experience does your partner enjoy sharing with you the most?
- Does your partner love or hate PDA?
- If your partner could take you on an intimate, romantic vacation, where would they choose to go?

Coupons

What you need:

Scissors

Optional:

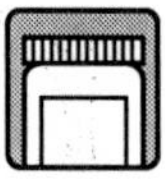

Peanut Butter

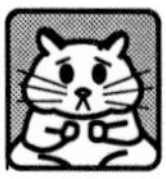

Hamster

How to Play:

When you get presented with one of these coupons, you are required to do what's on them for your partner!

I will let you

Sleep In

Undisturbed, on a weekend.

Expires: Never

Good for one session of

Cuddle Time

Expires: Never

I will make you

Breakfast in Bed

Expires: Never

One Idea a Day

What you need:

Paper

Pencil

Optional:

Whoopie Cushion

How to Play:

Spice up your sex life by doing one sexy thing each day.

1 In the middle of the night, wake your partner with a little oral surprise.

2 When you wake up, say, "I just had the sexiest dream." When they ask you to describe it, show them instead.

3 Write out a porn script, then act it out together.

4 After your partner goes to sleep, compose a steamy letter with things like "When I think about you doing blank, I get so turned on..." and put it someplace they will discover it in the morning.

5 Have sex with lights on and eyes wide open to connect on a whole new level.

6 Let your partner choose a sexy outfit for you to wear. Just the act of dressing for them, outfit or lingerie, will turn them on.

7 Take turns playing photographer. Even if you delete the photos at the end, it is a huge turn-on.

8 In public, whisper your fantasy or what you would like to do to your partner and let them stew in the thought until you get home. Have the stage set.

---

9 Fool around – but don't go all the way. NOT having sex can be a huge turn on.

---

10 Leave an invitation for lunch somewhere they will find it. Show up for lunch wearing a "sexed up" version of your everyday clothes. Let the lunch date be foreplay, and promise to finish the date that night.

---

11 Exchange your bedside lightbulbs with red ones to give the room a sexy glow.

---

12 Move to foot of the bed as things get heated. See how much one small change can heighten the sensations.

---

13 Wear his white dress shirt to bed with nothing underneath. Then get creative with a couple of his ties.

---

14 Take a swig of their favorite alcohol in the kitchen, then give them a seductive kiss as you saunter off to the bedroom. The taste of their favorite drink will have them intoxicated with love.

---

15 Challenge your partner to the world's quickest quickie.

---

16 Show your dominant side. Tie your partner's hands together with a silky scarf, tease them with no mercy with your lips and tongue. Playfully pull their hair to let them know who's in charge.

17 Create a private drive-in by watching a sexy flick on the portable DVD player in the car. Let the seats recline and the windows steam up.

---

18 Draw an imaginary line down the center of the bed. Get as wild as you can without crossing into each other's side.

---

19 Give your partner a gift certificate to a sexy novelty store. Tell them they can buy you anything they want you to wear (toys included). Shopping for the items can turn out to be serious foreplay.

---

20 Shower together at night with only a single candle glowing. The decreased visibility heightens the sense of touch. You'll be lucky to make it out of the bathroom for this round.

---

21 Watch a movie with your partner, but make it your goal to watch the entire thing. Slyly seduce each other with gentle touches, rubbing and kisses here and there. Hang in there until the movie is over and you are both ready to explode!

---

22 Create a Seductive Scavenger Hunt by making a list of sexy stuff for your partner to find or do by the end of the day.

---

23 Mirror, Mirror- Touch, kiss, and lick different areas of your partner's body, while they simultaneously touch, kiss, and lick you in exactly the same way.

---

24 Pour peppermint schnapps in your belly button. Have him sip it. Then have him kiss your breasts and blow on the spots he kissed. The peppermint schnapps and air combine for a cool sensation that heightens arousal.

---

25 Go out to dinner, and during the meal only talk about your sexual fantasies. Being surreptitious about your sexuality in public will be a turn-on for you both.

26 Do some "window" shopping at adult-toy websites. Pick out items that you both would enjoy experimenting with in the bedroom, then maybe purchase one if you're feeling adventurous!

---

27 Pick a day when you know the time your partner will be home. Before they get there, start baking their favorite treat wearing nothing but an apron. They'll be surprised and turned on when they arrive, plus they'll have a tasty dessert waiting for them after your round of hanky-panky.

---

28 Next time your partner is playing a video game, challenge them to a round. Every time you score in the game, take off a piece of clothing. Turning something so normal into an erotic event will make them forget all about the game.

---

29 Give each other tattoos - fake ones, that is. Buy body paint or use chocolate syrup and paintbrushes to draw, write or just smear the substances all over each other. Take a couples shower afterward to wash off the gunk and get down to business.

---

30 Become strangers for a night. Meet separately at a bar or coffee shop, and try to pick each other up. You'll bring back feelings from the beginning of your relationship while creating some suspenseful foreplay. If you want to kick it up a notch, rent a hotel room afterward instead of going home.

Turn watching a movie at home into something a little more: dim the lights, light some candles, strip down to your skivvies, and give each other hand or foot massages.

Sexual Bucket List

What you need:

Pencil

Optional:

Frozen Hot Dog

Cattle Prod

How to Play:

Create a risqué to-do list by coming up with various sexual activities you want to do before you die! Check them off with your partner as you accomplish them. Need some examples to get you started? How about: having a threesome; making love in a romantic travel spot, like Hawaii; partaking in a sexy boudoir photo shoot; or joining the Mile-High Club? The possibilities are endless.

Goal	Target Date	Done!
1.		
2.		
3.		
4.		
5.		
6.		
7.		

8.		
9.		
10.		
11.		
12.		
13.		
14.		
15.		
16.		
17.		
18.		
19.		
20.		

Guys, this one's for you: next time you go to the movies, use the "popcorn trick" on your partner. This is when you cut a hole in the bottom of the popcorn bowl, stick your wang through it, then wait for them to reach in for popcorn, but unknowingly get a surprise with their treat!

21.		
22.		
23.		
24.		
25.		
26.		
27.		
28.		
29.		
30.		
31.		
32.		
33.		
34.		
35.		

Answers

Pretty much sums it up.

What's Your Definition?

From Page 16

1. b. Punching a woman in the back of the head during sex
2. a. Getting clippings of someone's pubes thrown in your face
3. c. The word "Cock", said with a Boston accent
4. a. The medical term for foreskin
5. b. A medical condition which involves suffocating and having painful spasms, like during a heart attack
6. a. To give the female genitals a sparkly makeover with crystals to enhance their appearance
7. a. The medical term for tailbone
8. c. A false statement
9. a. A person who collects stamps
10. b. A person who can speak multiple languages
11. c. A species of turtle
12. a. A small town in Sri Lanka
13. d. A lesbian practice where two women rub their vaginas together during sex
14. c. The skin on your elbows
15. b. A slang term for the act of masturbating

What's Your Sex IQ?

From Page 30

Give yourself 20 points for each correct answer:

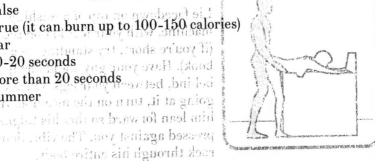

1. Yes
2. Women
3. False
4. True (it can burn up to 100-150 calories)
5. Car
6. 10-20 seconds
7. More than 20 seconds
8. Summer

Wrestling Move or Sex Act?

From Page 58

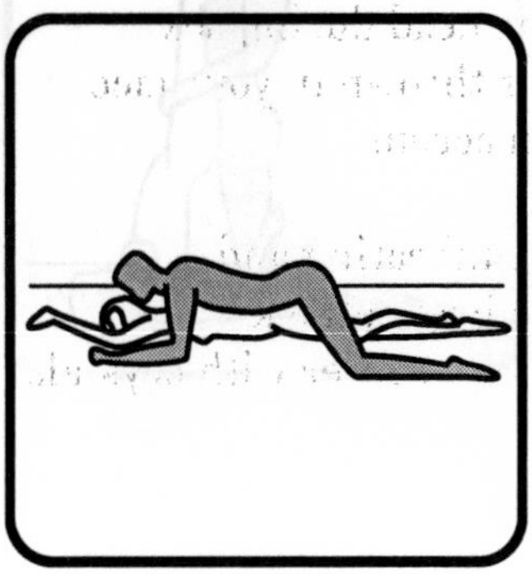

The Tight Squeeze

Lie down on your stomach and, keeping your legs straight, spread them slightly. Rest your arms by your side, or stretch them out in front of you. Have your guy stretch his body over yours, resting on his elbows so he doesn't place all his weight on you. He then positions his legs outside your legs. As he enters you, close your legs and cross them at the ankles.

The Pinwheel

You and your partner lie on your sides facing the same direction. First, you lower your crotch onto his, wrapping your legs around either side of his torso. Your arms should be stretched out behind you supporting your weight. He then encircles your waist with his legs and grips your upper thighs and thrusts gently.

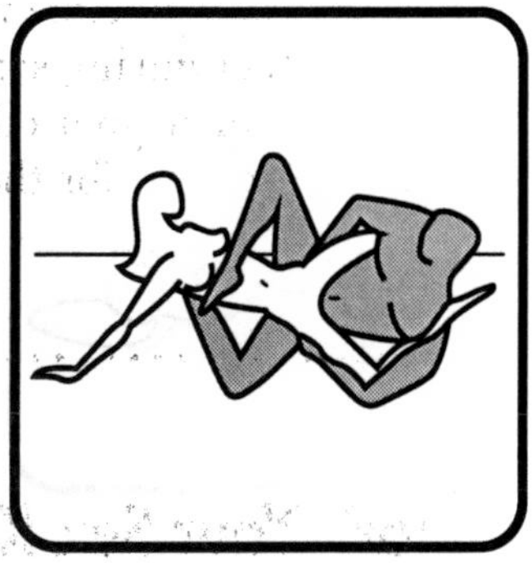

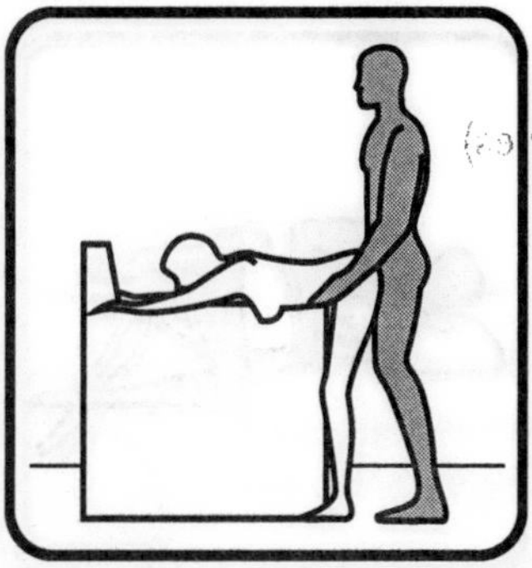

Mover and Shaker

Lie facedown on top of a washing machine, with your feet flat on the floor (if you're short, try standing on a phone book). Have your guy stand facing your behind, between your legs. Once you're going at it, turn on the machine. Have him lean forward so that his thighs are pressed against you. The vibrations will rock through his entire body.

The Head Game

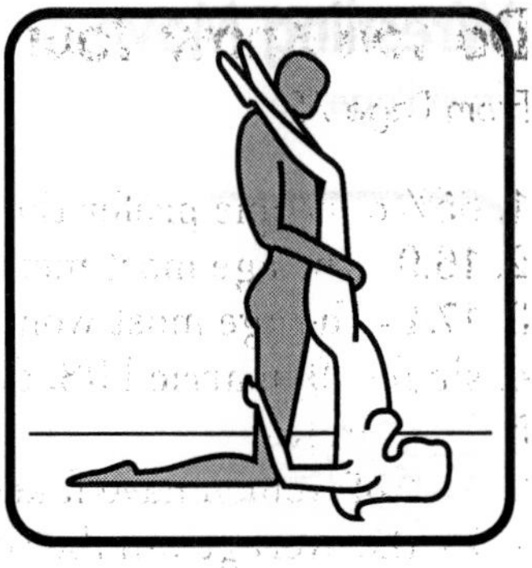

Lie flat on the ground face up. With your hands supporting your lower back, lift your legs and backside up so they're as perpendicular to the ground as you can get them. Have your man kneel before you, grab your ankles, and bring his knees to your shoulders. Then take his hands and ask him to hold your hips — that will steady you both. Hold his thighs for leverage and adjust so your genitals can join for some otherworldly upside-down action.

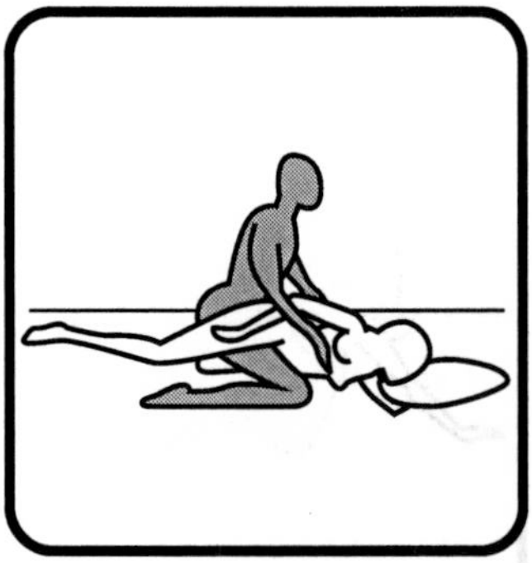

The Linguini

Lie on your side, putting a pillow under your head for extra support. Your man kneels directly behind your butt, leaning ever-so-slightly over your body. He should push one of his knees between your legs, positioning his body so he can penetrate you. He places one hand on your back to help support himself as he goes for the plunge. The key to your pleasure is keeping your limbs as limp as a noodle.

The Spider Web

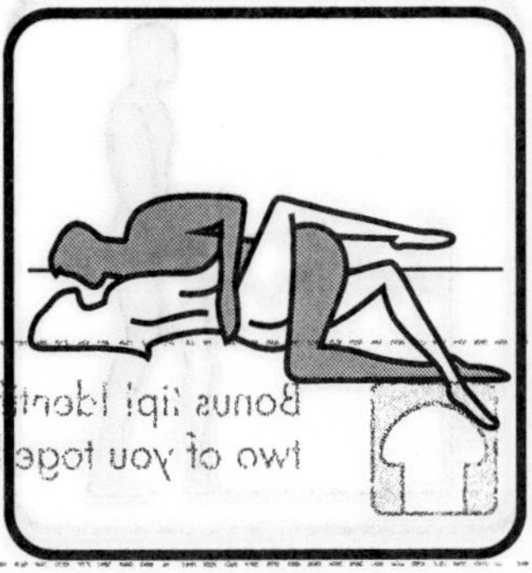

Both you and your guy lie on your sides, facing each other. Lean in close together and scissor your legs through his so you're superclose and he's deep inside you as he enters you. While thrusting, hold on to each other for leverage and ultimate friction.

Do You Know Your Sex Stats?

From Page 75

1. 65% of people prefer the light off
2. 16.9 - the age most men lose their virginity
3. 17.4 - the age most women lose their virginity
4. single 49; married 98; domestic couple 146
5. 20 minutes
6. 48% of women have faked an orgasm at least once
7. 7 - the average number of sexual partners for men
8. 4 - the average number of sexual partners for women
9. 7.4 minutes
10. 54% of men think about sex several times a day
11. 4% of men think about sex less than once per month
12. 48% of women want regular sex after four years of marriage

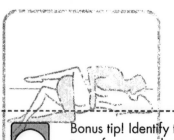

Bonus tip! Identify that one pivotal event that brought the two of you together. Celebrate that event every year.

Also by LoveBook™:

The Original "LoveBook™"
Create a custom gift book listing all of the reasons you love someone...we print it, bind it & ship it.

The Activity Book for Couples
Whether you are just dating or have been together for 50 years, these fun games and drawing activities are sure to bring laughter to your day!

The Romantic Coupon Book
A fun, romantic coupon book for anyone in love. This humorous coupon book will give your lover discounts and freebies that will keep you occupied for months! Contains 22 beautifully illustrated coupons.

The Bucket List for Couples
An exciting book to help couples come up with a list of goals that you'd like to achieve together. It includes categories, goal ideas, and pages to document your completed goals. A great way to spend time with your significant other while accomplishing amazing things.

The Marriage Advice Journal
Put all the words of wisdom from family and friends on how to make the most of marriage into one convenient book. This book make a great wedding or shower gift.

The Quiz Book for Couples
Think you know everything there is to know about your significant other? Put your knowledge to the test with this fun book of questions for every aspect of your relationship. It's a great way to learn more about your partner while engaging in a little healthy competition!

All of these titles and more can be found at
www.LoveBookOnline.com

About LoveBook™:

We are a group of individuals who want to spread love in all its forms. We believe love fuels the world and every relationship is important. We hope this book helps build on that belief.

CPSIA information can be obtained at www.ICGtesting.com
Printed in the USA
BVOW071258250712
296130BV00001B/370/P

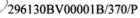

9 781936 806430